Advance Praise for
Transformed by Postpartum Depression

From her mini-van based research office, Dr. Walker Karraa has forged the future for maternal mental health. Her provocative book, Transformed by Postpartum Depression, *will challenge and change clinicians, researchers, and the public. Finally, the paradigm of PPD has been broadened to include trauma and the human condition. She has exposed a missing piece of the postpartum puzzle. Thank you, Walker!*

—Jane Honikman, MA, Founder, Postpartum Support
International

Walker Karraa has achieved greatness in the PPD community with her emphasis on trauma, transformation, and personal growth. What makes Transformed by Postpartum Depression *so uniquely powerful is that Karraa stands in the face of preconceived notions and challenges them with the stories and voices of real women who speak the truth and deserve to be heard. The conviction of these experiences holds tremendous healing power on behalf of the PPD woman seeking support as well as valued wisdom for the clinician who is accompanying this journey.*

—Karen Kleiman, MSW, Founder & Director, The
Postpartum Stress Center; Author, Therapy and the Postpartum Woman

The beauty of Dr. Karraa's book, Transformed by Postpartum Depression, *is that it is written not only for clinicians, but also for women who have suffered through postpartum depression. This book will provide much needed hope for mothers in the throes of this devastating mood disorder. The powerful narratives included in this book provide the readers with an insider's view of how mothers have been transformed by postpartum depression.*

—Cheryl Tatano Beck, DNSc, CNM, FAAN, Professor, School of Nursing, University of Connecticut

This book not only gives incredible insight into the raw and exquisitely agonizing truth about the experience of PPD, but it takes the concept and outcomes of treatment to a new, unexplored level. My clients have taught me over the last 20 years that PPD is indeed a traumatic, life stopping, and life altering experience that is not easily forgotten. Being inextricably intertwined with birth, a supposedly "blessed event," PPD shatters expectations and lives, and like a hurricane, blows women to pieces. Going beyond healing, Dr. Karraa explores concepts of resilience and taking women beyond simply surviving into thriving in their re-creation of a new self. This book takes a critical examination of a new direction in the field of PPD to help women create a new life through the process of healing, finding meaning and hope, and rebuilding.

—Pec Indman EdD, MFT, Author, Beyond the Blues

I found Walker Karraa's book an intelligent analysis of the debilitating process of postpartum depression and the significant impact it had on the lives of women and those close to them. It was sensitively written with elements of intense sympathy, empathy, and consideration for the courageous narratives which permeate throughout the book. Powerful personal thoughts were shared on the helplessness of suicidality and the need for something more than the superficiality of talk, but instead about the need for a solution and the hope that they would eventually improve. Walker's book offers a specific insight into the plight of mothers who have suffered from postpartum depression, and the cathartic, emotional journey they had to take to seek the peace they deserved. I really enjoyed reading the book and found it captured the elements of PPD in a very interesting and sensitive fashion.

Dr Jane Hanley, Past President of the International Marcé Society for Perinatal Mental Health, Hon Senior Lecturer in Primary Care, Public and Mental Health, College of Human and Health Sciences, Swansea University, Swansea, Wales

Transformed by Postpartum Depression

Women's Stories of Trauma and Growth

Walker Karraa, PhD

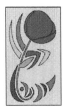

Praeclarus Press, LLC
www.PraeclarusPress.com

Praeclarus Press, LLC
2504 Sweetgum Lane
Amarillo, Texas 79124 USA
806-367-9950
www.PraeclarusPress.com

DISCLAIMER

The information contained in this publication is advisory only
and is not intended to replace sound clinical judgment or individ-
ualized patient care. The author disclaims all warranties, whether
expressed or implied, including any warranty as to the quality,
accuracy, safety, or suitability of this information for any particular purpose.

ISBN: 978-1-939807-21-2

Cover Design: Ken Tackett
Acquisition & Development: Kathleen Kendall-Tackett
Copy Editing: Chris Tackett
Layout & Design: Todd Rollison
Operations: Scott Sherwood

Dedication

This book is dedicated to my participants.

I have come

To drag you out of yourself

And take you into my heart.

I have come

To bring out the beauty

You never knew you had

And lift you like a prayer,

To the sky.

—Rumi

Table of Contents

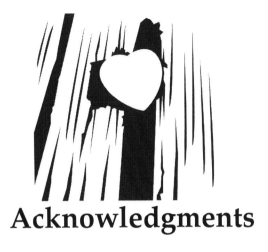

Acknowledgments

In addition to the extraordinary contributions of the 20 women who participated in my original research, I would like to acknowledge those who have offered additional support and assistance.

My dissertation committee members, Dr. Dorit Netzer and Dr. Kathleen Kendall-Tackett, offered critical guidance and expertise to my doctoral research.

I would like to give special acknowledgment to the chair of my dissertation, Dr. Mark McCaslin. Dr. McCaslin has never wavered in his support of my work and the continued development of the wisdom of wonder.

I would also like to thank the professionals who participated in interviews for this book, Cheryl Tatano Beck, Jane Shakespeare-Finch, Karen Kleiman, and Jane Honikman. I would like also acknowledge Richard Tedeschi for facilitating permission for me to use the Posttraumatic Growth Inventory.

I would like to thank my editor and friend, Meghan Pinson, and my transcriber, Trinitie Kedrowski, for their dedication and commitment to this work, and Praeclarus Press, for their work with me on this project.

Finally, I would like to offer special acknowledgment to my husband, Tony, my son, Ziggy, and my daughter, Miles. They were there with me, day-in and day-out, offering encouragement, coffee, and patience. My beautiful boy and brilliant girl—my dear ones, I have loved you since time began and will love you forever more. Thank you for loving me.

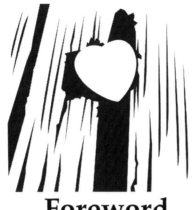

Foreword

Given that you are reading these words, dear reader, then I can safely assume the gravity of your purpose. Taking liberties, I would call it a rich and full purpose calling you to Dr. Walker Karraa's work with an intense reach for perspicuity. Perhaps you find yourself *Before*, seeking to quiet anxieties; or, *During*, where you are seeking answers, maps, directions… hope; or, *After*, where you empathically resonate with the stories of those transformed by postpartum depression. As well, I might count you as one who stands witness to this alchemy; a partner, friend, family… who is drawn to this *Krater[1]*, this fire, by friendship and love. Finally, I might count you as a professional–a healer whose purpose is to solve–to get to the heart of the matter. No matter your purpose, I will promise that you will find rich, full, and moving stories of being transformed by postpartum depression, insightful analyses for those standing

---

[1] Krater (mixing vessel), the vessel of spiritual transformation (Jung, 1963, p. 201)

witness, and solid research supporting an emerging theory of critical importance to the field.

Transformed by Postpartum Depression is a deeply rich, compelling journey. These women creatively engaged and transcended their "diagnosis," truly transforming themselves, their relationships, and their lives, finding self-empowerment within their personal creative journeys of healing. As a reader, it was humbling, revealing, and freeing. Freedom is what I find so often in my creative endeavors. And yet, just inside that freedom I find a peace of an unexplainable quality. *Transformed by Postpartum Depression* is this type of work, taking me to that very place of peace. Yes, that is it, there is a bridge between freedom and this sort of self-empathy that courageous creativity spans. Maslow speaks to this span of creativity as creative urges that guide us toward health and wholeness, finding creativity and this healthy wholeness to be one and the same. Natalie Rogers (1997) places the same healthy hope on creative expression as a force for therapeutic aims, stating that the creative is often therapeutic and that the therapeutic is often creative. And it becomes a short leap, pleasantly so, to find an enduring sense of freedom, of a deep and personal kind, emerging from such endeavors.

For me, the meta-problem considered for this work is, in fact, a consideration of freedom. The expression of a learning journey in the form of a grounded theory approach can, through its reflective and expressive qualities, foster a conversation between the personal and the social aspects of living and learning (Dominicé, 2000). Edel believed man "...reaches for the lives of others to assure himself of the commonalties of existence" (as cited by Lomask, 1984). According to Van-diver,

> Good biographies deal with the ways people faced living—tell how they met problems, how they coped with big and little crises, how they loved, competed, did the things we all do daily—and hence these studies touch familiar cords in readers (as cited by Kridel, 1998, p. 3).

And so, as you engage this profoundly moving and important work, you will experience this type of story, some astoundingly good analysis, and a practical and dynamic theory on personal transformation, personal creative healing, and finding redemptive freedom through postpartum depression. I certainly did.

Safe Journeys,

Mark McCaslin, PhD

List of Tables

List of Figures

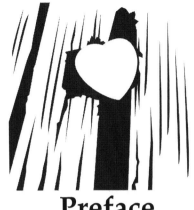

Preface

We must never forget that we may also find meaning in life even when confronted with a hopeless situation, when facing a fate that cannot be changed. For what then matters is to bear witness to the uniquely human potential at its best, which is to transform a personal tragedy into a triumph, to turn one's predicament into a human achievement.

—Victor Frankl (1959, p. 112)

In January 2011, I sat in a dissertation research class with about ten other doctoral students. The professor, Dr. Mark McCaslin, was asking that each of us describe what our dissertation topic might be. By the time it was my turn, I was speechless—stuck somewhere between forming the words and their very personal meaning. Dr. McCaslin looked at me for a moment and simply said, "I see you, Walker; and you know why you're here." I trusted him. I started talking… and didn't stop for the next three years. Dr. McCaslin became my doctoral advisor, and served as the chair of my dissertation committee.

What he saw in that moment was the clarity in my mind. He was right. I knew exactly what I wanted to study. I knew I wanted to study postpartum depression in a way that went beyond the suffering. By that time in my work as an advocate and writer, I had met so many women who described how postpartum depression (PPD) had changed them in powerful ways. I had met women who amazed me with their stories of survival, strength, and commitment to help others, despite unimaginable pain. They *had* suffered—greatly. But many, if not the majority, told me that the suffering served as a catalyst for significant personal change. Some change involved loss—women who never had another child, or had lost permanent custody of their children. Others had told me how PPD changed their goals or motivations in life—changing careers, starting non-profit organizations. The change women spoke of was profound. This change was my interest as a researcher. What was it about the nature of PPD to change the trajectory of a woman's life? How does a woman experience this change? What could we learn from women that might deepen our understanding of the pathology and its meaning in women's lives? Questions like these fueled my curiosity.

Truth be told, underlying my wonder was a constant voice telling me that there is more to women who suffer from a perinatal mood or anxiety disorder than just disease. I knew that science had only evidenced a part of the whole experience of PPD. We have benefitted tremendously from scientific inquiry into postpartum depression. We know more today than ever about the phenomenon of PPD. But then, why is it still so prevalent? And if we know that the vast majority of women who get PPD go undetected, what happens to them? Moreover, what about women who *do* suffer in view of science—those who score high on the screening instruments, those who meet diagnostic criteria (such that it is), who had risk factors known to increase likelihood of developing PPD, those who experienced the symptoms described in medical journals, those who undergo treatment that has been demonstrated to show some relief? What of them? Is that all there is? A laundry list of labels and recovery and then it's over?

I knew from my own experience that PPD is never over. It lingers. PPD marks a point on the map of one's life when things change forever. That point on the map is where I set up basecamp.

I spent nearly two years designing my study, researching the literature in the field, and passing through research protocol. I was ready to begin my interviews. I initially spoke with 37 women, and narrowed my final group to 20 women who had experienced PPD and reported that they considered their experience transformational. I did not define transformation or change—and they all asked! The answer was theirs to share; the story was theirs to tell.

In November 2012, I conducted my first formal research interview—in my minivan, parked in my driveway—the only private, quiet space I had as a mom/researcher/doctoral student. I spoke with for nearly 90 minutes. For the next two months, I got in and out of my minivan 19 more times, gathering over 25 hours of audio taped interviews.

I only asked four questions, designed carefully beforehand. Four questions were carefully chosen to invite descriptions of the experience of transformation through PPD, and the process of transformation through PPD. For the next nine months, I analyzed all 328 pages of their transcribed answers, using specific research methods called grounded theory (Appendix 1). Within a very short time, the experiences of 20 different women I am about to introduce had common themes that repeated over and over for all women. What stood out almost immediately was that transformation through PPD was a *long* journey.

- *Sienna*, a 28-year-old marketing communications specialist and mother of one, had experienced PPD five months prior to our interview. Sienna stated, "My process of transformation through postpartum depression, it's been a very long road, but I think in the end it has been transformational."

- *Skye*, a 39-year-old professional counselor who experienced PPD with both children, described, "I didn't really come back very quickly. It took a really long time. And it really colored how I felt about myself."

- *Stephanie*, a 29-year-old paralegal experienced PPD following the birth of her first child, approximately one year prior to the interview stated that, "I have come a long way."

- *Helena*, a 43-year-old mental-health therapist who experienced PPD following the births of both of her daughters 12 years prior to our talking, PPD was described in this way:

  It was like a slow earthquake that, that had big shocks, and smaller shocks, but it was undermining the structural integrity of my identity as a person at the time until I could kind of regroup, and build a different foundation.

- *Beatrice*, a 43-year-old psychologist and prenatal yoga instructor, also experienced PPD with both of her children, approximately six years before the time of the interview. She began:

  First of all, it was long, I would say. It wasn't something that happened very quickly—I wouldn't call it an extended postpartum depression, but it certainly wasn't short.

- *Haley*, age 35, a full-time financial analyst, experienced PPD following the birth of her second child, 18 months prior to the interview. She reflected, "I would say it took a while for me to kind of feel like myself again. I would say at least a year."

- *Georgia*, a 42-year-old former documentary producer and current psychotherapist (clinical social worker), has two children and experienced PPD following the birth of her first child. Georgia, when describing her sense of the speed of the transformation process, stated, "Overall the trajectory was, like, kind of slow and subtle."

- *Diana*, a 38 year old full-time student, experienced PPD approximately two years prior to our interview, following the birth of both of her children, who were born only 11 months apart. From Diana's perspective:

  It was a slow progression getting better over time. I tried taking control of little things. I controlled what I could, but I still was completely out of control. And, I tried, and I tried, and I tried. I tried "fake it until you make it" as long as I could. I definitely came out of it in baby steps.

- *Janis*, a 32-year-old master's level social-service professional, experienced PPD after the birth of her daughter, 10 months prior to the interview. Janis recounted:

  I think it took me a while, that awareness of the parts of me that were transforming. I think for a while I really—I externalized it. For a while and especially the first couple of months, I felt like it was something happening to me. So it took a while to shift.

- *Morgan*, a 48-year-old financial industry profession-al, had experienced PPD following the birth of her daughter nearly seven years prior to the interview. Morgan shared:

  It wasn't until I was totally out of the fog that I realized, "Wow, I just experienced postpartum depression."

- *Dana*, a 40-year-old mother of three, and adjunct university instructor and public-health graduate student, experienced PPD following the birth of her second and third children, approximately six years prior to the interview. Dana wrote a book about her experiences, noting:

  Yeah, after I wrote my book and released it, and did a few activities around that. It was kind of like that's how I made peace with it and I moved on.

- *Mindy*, a 45-year-old architectural lighting profes-sional, experienced PPD following the birth of her second child, nearly three years prior to the inter-view. Her completion of a photography project about PPD nearly a year after her experience sig-naled transformation in this way:

  It wasn't until I did my photography project, where I was able to, I think, fully, positively transform in my life and move forward because I realized at that point I didn't have to be stuck in these feelings, that that was part of my life, part of my pregnancy, part of my childbirth experience, but it didn't have to define me as a person.

- **Faith**, a 48-year-old volunteer and mother of three, experienced PPD following each of her births, slightly more than 13 years ago:

My first postpartum depression lasted with the anxiety, approximately 15 months. I was very young; I was 22 when I gave birth to my first son. My second son was born when I was 26, and we were in a place physically and financially that was better than when we were so young with our first son. Then we waited nine years after the birth of the middle son to have my third son. I think what blew me away about that experience is I thought I had it under control. My support system fell through, which began with my OB. It was quite scary. It took me 13 years to sign up to be able to volunteer to lead a postpartum support group. It took me that long to be able to be in a place in my head, and with me educating myself with resources, to feel confident enough to be able to help other women.

- **Sandy**, a 32-year-old social media professional, experienced PPD following the birth of her first and second child, shared:

Once you become depressed, you have to fight back to not only who you are, but you kind of have to let go of who you are and figure out who you are. And that, in and of itself, is very transformational because you're letting go of who you used to be because you're no longer that person. You're now a mother and you have this child and you're now battling a mental illness, which you may or may not have experience with prior to having given birth. You've got that, and then you're trying to figure what all of this makes you, all at the same time. So yeah, I think overall it's an extremely transformational process. I don't think I've talked to a single person ever who doesn't see it as such.

- *Karen*, a 30-year-old public health professional in a state agency, had experienced PPD two years prior to the interview. For Karen, her transformation was described in this way:

  Sure, well it was real slow. I mean I guess in the long run it feels fast, I guess, because it was only two years ago that it happened. But it definitely felt slow during the process, right? I was diagnosed at around six weeks postpartum. I'm almost two years out. So I say that my transformation is still happening. I say that the initial transformation was just me coming to the realization that I could ask for help, that that was an okay thing.

- *Vicki*, a 41-year-old advocate for a childhood tumor foundation, experienced PPD following the birth of her son, only a year before our interview. Vicki's description echoes the sense of recovery as having one speed, and the journey feeling long.

Even though I got help immediately, it was a long journey of getting better. But it was definitely hard.

- *Paula*, a 37-year-old quality professional and mental-health blogger, shared that a particularly difficult moment led to her realization of transformation sometime later:

I did have a really rough couple of weeks there, just because in one of my more frustrated moments, I had told my husband that, "You need to take her because I'm afraid I might hurt her." I was just frustrated. She wouldn't nurse, she wouldn't settle down, and at that point my husband didn't tell me until this incident happened several months ago, he said, "When you said that, I started making plans to what I would do if something happened." He never wanted to leave me alone with the girls and he made plans on what he would do if he thought I was a danger to myself or the girls. Hearing that made me realize I was really, really struggling. But I'm better and I can use my experience and my voice to help other moms realize they're not alone and it's okay to talk about these scary things because the more we talk about them, the more people can be educated and hopefully we can prevent tragedies before they happen.

- *Jamie*, 31-year-old high-level software tester in the technical industry, experienced PPD following the birth of her son, only two years prior to the interview. For Jamie, transformation through PPD was signaled in this way:

One thing that's been extremely transformational was a year after he was born, when my son's birthday came around, I went back to my therapist. One of the things I said was, "You know, I just hated that hospital because all these people were touching me without my permission and it just felt so awful." And she said, "Well has that ever happened to you before? Has anybody done that to you before?" I was raped 14 years ago and I never told anybody and right then, I told her.

- **Betsy**, 35, an actress, author and mother of two, began her long journey with PPD early after her birth:

You know while I was in it, obviously it was all negative, but I think in the long term I actually see it as what made my transformation into a mother complete because what I learned so early on was that there's no way to be perfect. There was going to be a lot that wasn't in my control and a lot that I didn't understand. So, you know, time has given me the luxury of being able to see it that way.

- **Anna**, a 37-year-old professional fundraiser, and now stay-at-home mother, described her journey as a reflection on a specific change in her appearance:

When I was talking to my husband about this interview and that I was going to talk to you, he said, "You have to tell her about the earrings." When I graduated from high school, my grandparents gave me this beautiful pair of pearl earrings, and I wore them every day and by saying I wore them every day, I literally mean those were the only pair of earrings I ever wore. Being a high school senior through [to] when my son was born, I wore those pearl earrings every day. I just considered it part of my identity. They were kind of a signature item. But now I wear different jewelry all the time.

Anna was changed through her experience of PPD, just as each of these women was changed by PPD. The stories they share in this book tell us what we need to know, what we must know about PPD—it is a force of nature that has the power to destroy an entire life. The struggle to survive the damage of PPD can be a long journey of isolation, fear, terrifying confusion, and life-threatening peril. And those who live to tell the tale? *Call them Ishmael.*

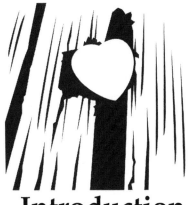

Introduction

Society does not want to hear the reality of the experience, which is that the experience of having a baby and learning to become a mother are a total experience and a life-altering event. It can be a time of significant growth and self-awareness. It is a time when many women are able to reassess and become self-aware, self-confident, and authentic.

(Beck & Driscoll, 2006, p. 59)

Public knowledge of PPD has been informed through science and media. While the awareness campaigns have succeeded in bringing PPD to the attention of society, postpartum depression remains a critical public health concern. Interestingly, depression is the second most common cause of hospitalization for all women in the U.S.; the first being childbirth (Blenning & Paladine, 2005; Gold & Marcus, 2008). Current estimates are that in the United States, postpartum depression (PPD) impacts 15% to 25% of women annually (Gavin et al., 2005; Keyes & Goodman, 2006). The World Health Organization (WHO) has suggested that global prevalence rates for women suffering from PPD are as high as 34% to 55% (WHO, 2003), with a sevenfold increase in the risk of psychiatric hospitalization for all women following childbirth (Harlow, Vitonis, Sparen, Cnattinguis, Joffe, & Hultman, 2007).

Obstetricians have finally acknowledged postpartum depression. In 2009, Dr. Gerald F. Joseph Jr. became the first president of the American College of Obstetricians and Gynecologists (ACOG) to make his presidential initiative PPD (Joseph, 2009). Increased awareness from ACOG has been underscored by further research reporting PPD as one of the most common serious complications of childbirth (Bruce et al., 2008). For example, Bruce et al. (2008) studied 24,481 pregnancies among 21,011 women and found that mental health was one of the most common complications of childbirth. Evidence such as this continues to proliferate in medical journals. Still ACOG policy states that there is not enough of it to mandate mental health screening for women in pregnancy and postpartum. Two steps forward, one step back.

Another example of progress *not* progressing can be found in prevalence rates. Prevalence is a measurement of the amount of a disease that occurs in a population of people at a particular point in time. While strides have been made to increase awareness of PPD in medical sciences over the last two decades, prevalence rates remain relatively unchanged. For example, consider that in 1996, O'Hara and Swain published the landmark meta-analysis of 59 studies to gauge how often PPD occurs in the general population. They found a prevalence rate of 13%. As recently as 2008, the Centers for Disease Control and Prevention (U.S. Centers for Disease Control [U.S. CDC], 2008) analyzed data from 17 states in the United States and reported prevalence rates of 10% to 15%. In the span of nearly 20 years, prevalence rates for PPD have remained unchanged. With all of the research, prevention campaigns, blogs, and media attention (good and bad) paid to PPD in the span of two decades—and we still have the same number of women getting PPD. What are we missing?

One clue could be the report that as many as 50% of women with PPD go untreated (Mental Health America: Substance Abuse and Mental Health Services Administration [SAMHSA], 2009). A second clue might be that while the most common treatment intervention is psychopharmacology, some women are resistant to taking medication without being offered a range of nonmedical treatment options. Additionally, we might consider that PPD affects poor women more, with PPD prevalence rates reported as high as 48% of women living in poverty (Knitzer, Theberge, & Johnson, 2008). Another clue to the steady prevalence rates could be that beliefs and attitudes regarding mental health in the postpartum period have been reported to be significant barriers to treatment (Bilszta, Ericksen, Buist, & Milgrom, 2005; Dennis & Chung-Lee, 2006; Goodman, 2009). With all of this evidence about PPD, we have yet to fully understand the dynamics involved in experiencing PPD.

Jane Hanley, perinatal mental illness researcher and 2012-2013 President of the International Marcé Society for Perinatal Mental Health, has offered this important insight:

> At the present time, Western society has construct-ed perinatal mental health within a medical frame-work, and there is no doubt that the recognition and treatment of the conditions have been very benefi-cial in some instances. Whilst there is no intention to denigrate the contribution medicine makes to the treatment of this condition, the construction of mothers' mental health within a critical framework is claimed by some to provide an alternative option for intervention. This option illustrates how exter-nalizing the effects of the condition may help wom-en to recover more quickly from their experiences (Hanley, 2009, p. 193).

Hanley's (2009) suggestion is a bold one: a paradigm of perinatal mental illness that includes science and women—a framework of maternal health that makes room for women to externalize their experiences as part of a broad spectrum of normal. I wholeheartedly agree. We need both medicine and mothers to create the future of maternal mental health.

Towards a Positive Psychology Model of Post-partum Depression

There is good research bringing mothers together with science: namely, the qualitative research about the lived experience of PPD, the work of Cheryl Beck and others, is some of the best research we have because the women themselves to describe PPD. The amount of qualitative research pales in comparison to more traditional, and therefore more funded, quantitative research. Furthermore, the early qualitative studies are defined by the medical model of disease-based pathology and suffering. Previous studies have not asked women about the process, results, or meaning given to that suffering.

Existential psychologist and Holocaust survivor Victor Frankl (1959), learned through his own direct experience of severe torture, suffering, and loss, that part of the essence of the human experience is our capacity to find meaning in living through tragedy. He said, "In some way, suffering ceases to be suffering at the moment it finds meaning" (p. 113). Transforming suffering into personal growth is a hallmark of human potential, occupying an important place in positive and transpersonal psychology (Braud & Anderson, 1998). However, there are no positive psychology studies about PPD, or any perinatal mental illness. The closest we have gotten to integrating science, medicine, and women's experience in our research is, arguably, breast cancer. In breast cancer research, all schools of medicine, psychology, sociology, feminism, and traumatology have examined and therefore expanded our understanding of both the disease and the survival of the disease.

Limitations of Previous Models

Here is the critical missing link. Humanistic and existential psychology, that have long since embraced the human experience of suffering as a core function of personal growth, have not yet considered suffering of perinatal mental illness as a research subject. To date, what we know about PPD is medically based because that is the field that has treated it firsthand. Obstetrics, midwifery, nursing, and medical psychiatry have produced the largest amount of data on PPD. It is no wonder then, that our understanding of PPD, to a large extent, is based on a disease model.

It is interesting to note that large health organizations have begun to address the need for new paradigms of both physical and mental health that move beyond disease-based models. Namely, the definitions of health and disease are being revised. For example, the World Health Organization (WHO, 2001) defined *physical health* as "a state of complete physical, mental, and social well-being, and not merely the absence of disease or infirmity" (p. 1). Additionally, the WHO (2001) defined *mental health* as "a state of well-being in which the individual realizes his or her own abilities, can cope with the normal stresses of life, can work productively and fruitfully and is able to make a contribution to his or her community" (p. 1).

More recently, the Centers for Disease Control and Prevention (2009) defined *health* as "a state of complete physical, mental, and social well-being and not just the absence of sickness or frailty" (2009, p. 1). Another example, the United States Department of Health and Human Services (U.S. Department of Health and Human Services [U.S. DHHS], n.d.) *Healthy People 2020* report, suggested care providers and researchers use a matrix of wellness that would "assess the positive evaluations of people's daily lives—when they feel very healthy and satisfied or content with life, the quality of their relationships, their positive emotions, resilience, and realization of their potential" (p. 16). The Institute of Medicine (IOM, 2011) has endorsed the *Healthy People 2020* (U.S. DHHS, n.d.) initiatives to examine topics of social determinants of health, and health-related quality of life and well-being in policy and practice.

So where is a mother with PPD in all of this policy, theory, and research about quality of life, contentment, satisfaction, and realizing her own potential? Invisible. That is the purpose of this book. This book puts wisdom to work in the world of maternal mental health. It describes the ways women who are mothers survive the suffering of a pathology, PPD, and continue to grow and create lives that feel healthy, content, and guided toward their greatest human potential. In this way, this book is a call to re-search the impact of PPD on a woman's life, and re-view her abilities to change and grow through it.

Description of the Book

In *Chapter 1, Postpartum Depression,* I outline current definitions and research regarding prevalence, risk factors, and the effects of PPD on women and children. This chapter provides an important backdrop to the rest of the book as it explains the context that each and every woman in my research lived her experience, setting the stage for the description of PPD as both traumatic and transformational. *Chapter 2, Before PPD,* describes the first dimension of transformation through PPD as women reported being unprepared. *Chapter 3, During PPD:* **I Was Shattered (and No One Picked Up the Pieces)**, describes the traumatic impact of PPD and the tragic failure of providers to address, treat, or acknowledge the symptoms. *Chapter 4, Ending PPD: Getting Better,* describes the ways women worked as agents to find the help they critically needed. *Chapter 5, After PPD: I Was a Different Person,* describes how women experienced the transformation in their lives, relationships, and professional interests. *Chapter 6, Beyond PPD:* **Metamorphosis**, explains how women experienced transformative growth in the final dimension—where levels of growth surpassed resiliency or recovery. *Chapter 7, Trauma and Transformation,* reviews the current ideas regarding change and growth through adversity in order to hone in on the most accurate understanding of the trauma and transformation of PPD.

Chapter 8, Professional Perspectives, presents interviews I conducted with four experts in the field: Cheryl

Beck, Karen Kleiman, Jane Shakespeare-Finch, and Jane Honikman. The variety of expertise, experience, and opinion regarding viewing PPD as a traumatic life event is disparate and thought provoking. This chapter begins the cross-disciplinary dialogue regarding how we view women, PPD, trauma, treatment, and research. *Chapter 9, PPD Grows Up: New Reflections*, concludes the book with a circling back to the current view of PPD and the expanding conversation and paradigm that is offered in this book.

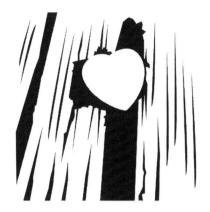

Chapter 1

Postpartum Depression

Some of the most powerful images of women and motherhood are those held by the professional disciplines which lay claim to a special expertise in the field of reproduction—namely, medical science, clinical psychiatry, and psychology.

(Anne Oakley, 1993, p. 19)

The images of PPD, as described by the professions that have studied it, create a mosaic of sorts. The picture of PPD that exists today is a collage of definitions, diagnoses, treatments, measurements, and theories considered by medical science, nursing, psychology, psychiatry, and to a lesser extent a small number of feminist theories from sociology. This chapter provides an overview of research that will help you understand the full impact of the experiences of transformation through PPD described in the following chapters. What is presented, therefore, in this chapter is the picture of PPD as defined by the professionals who have studied it.

What is Postpartum Depression?

The most powerful health institutions grapple with the language of PPD. The World Health Organization (WHO, 2009) defines PPD as "a clinical and research construct used to describe an episode of major or minor depression arising after childbirth" (p. 17). According to the American Psychiatric Association (APA, 2013), postpartum depression refers to a "nonpsychotic depressive episode that begins in the postpartum period" (p. 160). The word *postpartum* in both cases is used as an onset specifier for a diagnosis of Major Depressive Disorder (MDD). In other words from the medical standpoint, PPD is major depression that happens after childbirth.

What is Major Depressive Disorder (MDD)? It is the experience of five or more of the following symptoms present nearly every day, during the same two-week period: (a) depressed mood (sadness, hopelessness), (b) lack of interest or pleasure in all or most activities, (c) significant weight loss or weight gain, (d) insomnia or hypersomnia, (e) psychomotor agitation or retardation, (f) fatigue, (g) feelings of worthlessness or excessive or inappropriate guilt, (h) poor concentration, (i) recurrent thoughts of death, (j) recurrent suicidal ideation without a specific plan, or a suicide attempt or a specific plan for committing suicide. Symptoms are not attributable to other medical conditions, and are presented either by subjective report or observation of others (APA, 2013, pp. 160-161).

PPD symptoms are consistent with those in MDD (Preston & Johnson, 2009)—with one huge exception: motherhood. Women who have PPD are experiencing a full-blown episode of major depression in addition to the increased demands of caring for a newborn and recovering from childbirth. Leading PPD researcher, Michael O'Hara (2009) noted that:

Major depression creates suffering whether experienced in the postpartum period or at any other time in a woman's life. What makes depression so poignant for postpartum women is that childbirth is culturally celebrated and there is an expectation that new parents, especially mothers, will be joyful, if not tired, during this time. Moreover, the demands on a new mother are substantial and include providing 24-hour care for a newborn, often in the middle of the night, caring for older children, keeping up with normal household responsibilities, and often returning to work after a brief maternity leave. These burdens are often difficult to bear in normal circumstances and the difficulty of bearing them is exacerbated by the disability associated with depression symptoms (e.g., sad mood, loss of interest, motor retardation, difficulty concentrating) (p. 1259).

O'Hara's (2009) description resonates; PPD is different. It is an experience of psychiatric illness during a life event unlike any other: motherhood. However, in the eyes of medical science, PPD is still defined as an MDD that sometimes can occur in women after childbirth. When exactly is that? The window of time when the diagnosis can be given has been hotly debated. Since the first use of postpartum specifier in the DSM-III (APA, 1994), the timing was set at four weeks following the birth of a baby. Clinical experts have petitioned for expanding that time frame based on what they are seeing in their patients, that symptoms of PPD can arise three to six months after childbirth. The most recent DSM-5 (APA, 2013) extended the timing to six weeks. There will not be another DSM revision until 2020. How this translates for women is that the timing of their symptoms must fall within the first six weeks after having a baby if they are to meet the criteria for major depression with postpartum onset.

Bottom line, the only two medical manuals that describe physical and psychiatric illnesses do not have a specific diagnosis for PPD. How this translates for women and providers is important. When women have symptoms, there is no clear description for the care provider to consult, or a medical code to chart that communicates to other providers that she has PPD. Unpacking this a bit further, we can understand that the lack of a specific clinical diagnostic classification for PPD in the *Diagnostic and Statistical Manual of Mental Disorders-5* (DSM-5; American Psychiatric Association [APA], 2013) and the *International Classification of Dis-*

eases (ICD 10; WHO, 1992) reveals the lack of understanding of the phenomenon itself. Clearly we have a lot of work to do with regards to aligning our medicine with our mothers.

What PPD is NOT

A dangerous mixture of stigma and misunderstanding has led to a global association between the word "postpartum" and tragic cases involving infanticide. These cases receive significant media attention. Confusion in media reporting fuels devastating stereotypes that marginalize mothers, and creates powerful social obstacles to seeking help. Media reports misinterpreting the research regarding safety of psychiatric medication during pregnancy and postpartum can have dangerous implications for women who choose to discontinue medication without proper medical assessment. There is a significant absence of media reports regarding trauma in pregnancy and postpartum women, both in our military service women and the civilian population. There is an overwhelming sensationalist portrayal of perinatal psychosis that leads to infanticide, and relatively little reporting on the instances of perinatal suicide, self-harm, negative impact on children, or the new understanding of the role of bipolar disorder in the development of postpartum psychosis (Wisner et al., 2013).

What we do know is that there is a spectrum of psychological diagnoses during the perinatal period, ranging from the most mild, postpartum blues, to the most severe, postpartum psychosis (APA, 2013; Gavin et al., 2005; O'Hara & Segre, 2008). Postpartum blues is described as "mood lability, irritability, interpersonal hypersensitivity, insomnia, anxiety, tearfulness, and sometimes elation" (O'Hara, 2009, p. 1259). Postpartum blues, maternity blues, or "baby blues" (Bennett & Indman, 2011, p. 34) was introduced to the medical literature by Maloney (1952) as "third-day depression" (p. 21). Postpartum blues presents mild, time-limited symptoms of depression, such as irritability, mood swings, and tearfulness occurring soon after childbirth and resolving within 10 to 14 days following childbirth (O'Hara & Segre, 2008). Postpartum blues are reported to occur from 50% to 80% of mothers following childbirth (Beck, 2006; Moses-Kolko & Roth, 2004). Usually postpartum blues resolves itself without treatment (Moses-Kolko & Roth, 2004), but may be a risk factor for the more severe PPD (Beck, 2006; O'Hara & Segre, 2008).

At the other end of the spectrum of perinatal mental illness is the most severe, and life-threatening disorder: postpartum psychosis. Postpartum psychosis affects one to two women per 1,000 births globally, and while rare, it is an extremely severe postpartum mood disorder and is a psychiatric emergency that requires immediate medical attention.

Who Gets Postpartum Depression?

PPD has been shown to affect rural and low-income women disproportionately (Howell, Mora, Horowitz, & Leventhal, 2005; Jesse & Swanson, 2007; Knitzer et al., 2008;

Mora et al., 2009; Moses-Kolko & Roth, 2004; Segre, O'Hara, Arndt, & Stuart, 2007). Prevalence rates among African American, Hispanic, and Native American women may be underestimated. The influence of racial/ethnic disparities in care on the reporting of depressive symptoms has yet to be fully examined (Breslau, Kendler, Su, Gaxiola-Aguilar, & Kessler, 2005). Factors of discrimination, violence, poverty, stigma regarding mental health, preferential diagnosis among Caucasian women, compared to minority women, have been reported as contributors to women of color not seeking mental health care (Borowsky, Rubenstein, Meredith, Camp, Jackson-Triche, & Wells, 2000; Nadeem, Lange, Eddge, Fongwa, & Miranda, 2007).

A nationally representative study of pregnant women (N=3,051) determined that "non-white and Hispanic women without a history of mental health were less likely to report poor antepartum mental health" (Witt et al., 2010, p. 433). Other studies have suggested that ethnic underrepresentation in mental health research, less satisfaction with services received, or negative beliefs about treatment contribute to underestimating prevalence for minority women in the United States (Cooper et al., 2003; Diala et al., 2001; Miranda & Cooper, 2004; McGuire, Alegria, Cook, Wells, & Zaslavsky, 2006; Wang et al., 2005). Segre, O'Hara, and Losch (2006) examined race/ethnicity as a risk factor for depressed mood in late pregnancy and early postpartum period, reporting that African American women were significantly more likely to report depressed mood; while

Hispanic American women were significantly less likely to report being depressed. How could this be?

The majority of women giving birth in the United States are Latina (Hayes-Bautista, Hsu, Perez, & Kahramanian, 2003; U.S. Census Bureau, 2004). However, U.S. Hispanic mothers may be less likely to use mental health care services as compared to other minority women, regardless of income or insurance coverage (Vega, Kolody, & Aguilar-Gaxiola, 2001). Cerda (2003) reported that Latina mothers are three times less likely to use mental health care. Systemic barriers to treatment for Latinas may be so strong as to skew the prevalence rates altogether. In a study of Hispanic new mothers (N=218), Chaudron et al. (2005) reported 28% of mothers self-identified as needing help with depression since the birth of their baby, and less than half had discussed depression with their care provider. In other words, women knew they were ill, but didn't discuss it with their providers.

More recent studies of PPD for Latina women show promise. For example, Baker-Ericzen et al. (2012) experimented with a telemedicine intervention based on the Perinatal Mental Health model and demonstrated telephone intervention as feasible and acceptable intervention (Baker-Ericzen, Mueggenborg, Hartigan, Howard, & Wilke, 2008).

Global Prevalence

Our data on global rates of PPD demonstrate solid evidence that PPD is not culturally bound (Eberhard-Gran, Garthus-Nigel, Garthus-Nigel, & Eskild, 2010). In an early landmark study, Kumar (1994) presented strong findings that "there are no major differences in rates of postnatal depression in the few crosscultural comparisons that have so far been reported" (p. 256). In fact, WHO (2001) reported that for all women aged 15 to 44 years, major depression is second only to HIV/AIDS in terms of total disability. The Global Burden of Disease for women suffering from mental illness is profound. From a public health perspective, Almond (2009) reviewed the epidemiological literature reporting a global incidence rate "much higher than the quoted rate of 10% to 15%" (p. 221). In Italy, Banti et al. (2011) reported a period prevalence of 9.6% in a study of over 1,000 women. In a study of rates of PPD for 1,659 Arab women in Qatar, Bener, Gerber, and Sheikh (2012) reported a prevalence rate of 18.6% for PPD. In a Latin American study of 1,256 women, Wolf, De Andraca, and Lozoff (2002) reported prevalence rates at 35% to 50%. Fisher et al. (2012) examined the rates of PPD published in over 1,000 studies of PPD in low income countries, reporting an overall rate 19.8% —a much higher prevalence than high-income countries.

Risk Factors for PPD

What we know about PPD is that there are risk factors associated with increasing the chance of developing PPD. What is risk? Goodman and Dimidjian (2012) noted that:

> Risk is defined as a condition that increases the probability of developing a disorder. A risk factor necessarily precedes the onset of the disorder and is difficult to identify empirically, as prospective longitudinal designs are required. More research has focused on correlates of depression (that is, factors that tend to co-occur with depression rather than risk) (p. 532).

From this perspective, explanation of the risk factors experienced before and during pregnancy leads to a better understanding of the physical, psychological, and socioeconomic conditions associated with the probability of developing PPD. In an early meta-analyses, Beck (2001) analyzed 84 studies, with a combined total sample size (N = 3,000). She reported 13 predictors of postpartum depression as statistically significant, rated as being moderate or having a small effect size. The moderate risks reported were prenatal depression, childcare stress, life stress, social support, prenatal anxiety, marital dissatisfaction, depression history, infant temperament, and self-esteem (Beck, 2001). Recent literature bears this data out, and has produced a new understanding that many of the risk factors for PPD are found before and during pregnancy.

Maternal Age, Parity, and History of Mood or Anxiety Disorder

First-time mothers and mothers who are young have a higher risk of developing PPD (Borjesson et al., 2005; Records & Rice, 2007; U.S. CDC, 2008;Vesga-Lopez et al., 2008). Prior history of mental-health problems has been shown as a significant risk factor for the development of PPD (Bilszta et al., 2005; Borjesson et al., 2005; Johnstone, Boyce, Hickey, Morris-Yatees, & Harris, 2001; Josefsson et al., 2002; Lancaster et al., 2010; Marcus, Flynn, Blow, & Barry 2003; Mora et al., 2009; O'Hara & Gorman, 2004).

Depression during pregnancy has also been reported as a significant risk factor for the development of PPD (Beck, 2001; Goodman & Tully, 2009; Leigh & Milgrom, 2008). In a systematic review of all of the research to date, Gaynes et al. (2005) reported that 14.5% of women developed a new episode of major or minor depression in pregnancy. Wisner et al. (2001) reported that a woman who has had one episode of postpartum depression has a 25% chance of recurrence.

Obstetric Risk Factors

Women with a history of obstetric complications, such as stillbirth or miscarriage, are at increased risk of developing PPD (Forman, Videbech, Hedegaard, Salvig, & Secher, 2000; Johnstone et al., 2001; Josefsson et al., 2002; Rubertsson, Waldenstrom, & Wickberg, 2003). Unplanned or unwanted pregnancy has been demonstrated as a risk factor for PPD (Fisher et al., 2012; Lancaster et al., 2010; Lee et al.,

57

2007; Mora et al., 2009; Rich-Edwards et al., 2006; Ruberts-son et al., 2003). Depression during pregnancy increases the risk of poor birth outcomes, preterm birth, and low birth-weight (Rahman et al., 2003).

Psychosocial Risk Factors

Women with low self-esteem are at higher risk for PPD (Beck, 2001; Chaudron, 2001; Jesse & Swanson, 2007; Lee et al., 2007; Leigh & Milgrom, 2008). In addition, women without social support are also at higher risk (Jesse & Swanson, 2007; Lancaster et al., 2010; Lee et al., 2007; Leigh & Milgrom, 2008; Rubertsson et al., 2003; Rudnicki, Graham, Habboushe, & Ross, 2001; Westdahl et al., 2007). Non-part-nered or unmarried mothers are at increased risk for devel-oping PPD, as are mothers in unhappy partnerships or mar-riages (Henry, Beach, Stowe, & Newport, 2004; Lancaster et al., 2010; Lee et al., 2007; Marcus et al., 2003; Orr, 2004; Re-cords & Rice, 2007; Rich-Edwards et al., 2006). In a system-atic review, Fisher et al. (2012) reported that for pregnant and postpartum women in low- and lower-to-middle-in-come countries, psychosocial risk factors included (a) being unmarried; (b) lack of intimate partner support; (c) having hostile in-laws; (d) lack of emotional or practical support; and (e) intimate partner violence.

Socioeconomic and Cultural Risk Factors

Poverty has been associated with increased life stress and depression in the general population since the latter part of the 20th century (Holmes & Rahe, 1967). So it is no surprise that poor women are at higher risk. This has been reported extensively in the literature (Beck, 2001; Holzman et al., 2006; Jesse, Walcott-McQuigg, Mariella, & Swanson, 2005; Lancaster et al., 2010; Leigh & Milgrom, 2008; Marcus et al., 2006; Rubertsson et al., 2003; Vesga-Lopez et al., 2008; Westdahl et al., 2007). In a study with a large sample of postpartum women (N=4,332), Segre et al. (2007) reported income as the strongest predictor for PPD. Segre et al. (2007) also noted occupational prestige, marital status, and number of children were also significant predictors. Relative, rather than absolute, economic disadvantage was relevant, as noted by inclusion of the Wan et al. (2009) study reporting that not owning a car in Beijing is associated with a higher risk of common postpartum mood disorders.

The Combination of Risk Factors

The research regarding risk factors has demonstrated that PPD does not occur in isolation, but rather in "conjunction with a complex interplay of sociodemographic, biophysical, psychosocial, and behavioral factors" (Jesse & Swanson, 2007, p. 378). Previous history of mental health problems, maternal age, obstetric problems, unplanned pregnancies, lack of social support, violence in the home, and poverty have all been found as correlates to the development of PPD. The pathways through which these factors create risk in some, and not in others, have been of interest to the field of developmental psychopathology. Kendall-Tackett (2010) explained:

Women do not become mothers in a vacuum. They live in families, extended families, cultures, and societies. At each of these levels of social connection, mothers can be protected from or made more vulnerable to depression (p. 104).

What Are the Effects of PPD?

The research regarding effects of PPD on mothers and their infants has been substantial. I first offer a brief overview of the research on the effects of PPD on women. Secondly, I review some of the effects of PPD on infants and children.

Maternal Mortality

You may be surprised to learn that suicide is one of the leading causes of maternal mortality during the first year after childbirth (Chang et al., 2005; Copersino et al., 2005; Howard et al., 2011; Lindahl et al., 2005; Oates, 2003; Palladino et al., 2011). In an early study from the United Kingdom, Oates (2003) reported that of the total 378 incidences of maternal death (death within 42 days postpartum), between the years 1997 and 1999, suicide was the leading cause of death. More recently, the *2004 Confidential Enquiry into Maternal and Child Health* reported depression and obesity as the major causes of death in pregnant and postpartum women in the United Kingdom (Lewis, 2007).

A 2005 review of studies reported suicides accounting for 20% of deaths; and the percentage of mothers with thoughts of self-harm during pregnancy and postpartum ranged from 5% to 14% (Lindahl et al., 2005). Most recently, researchers analyzed the death records for women of reproductive age who died between 2003 and 2007, using the CDC's National Violent Death Reporting System (Palladino et al., 2011). The report stated that "the rates of pregnancy-associated homicide and suicide were each higher than mortality rates attributable to common obstetric causes" (Palladino et al., 2011, p. 1059). Moreover, 51% of the suicides occurred during the postpartum period. Victims were significantly more likely to be unmarried, Caucasian, or Native American. In 54% of the cases, intimate partner conflict contributed to suicide (Palladino et al., 2011).

Suicidal Ideation

The precursor to suicide, in most cases, is suicidal ideation, or intrusive thoughts of suicide, and the presence of major depression (Lewis & Drife, 2004; Lindahl et al., 2005; Perez-Rodriguez, Baca-Garcia, Oquendo, & Carlos, 2008; Wisner et al., 2013). Howard et al. (2011) examined suicidal ideation in a large (N = 4,150) sample of postpartum women using the Edinburgh Postnatal Depression Scale (EPDS) (Cox et al., 1987). Nine percent of 4,150 women reported some suicidal ideation, and 4% reported thoughts of harming themselves occurring sometimes or quite often.

Given that the majority of women who get PPD go untreated or undetected, and the rates of completed suicides in the postpartum period remains relatively low, it is safe to argue that we have little idea as to how frequently women experience suicidal ideation postpartum. What does it do to a woman to be a mother of an infant and want to die? How are those thoughts while caring for a newborn resolved, recovered, or remembered years after? For the mothers in my study, there was a shocking relationship between suicidal ideation and PPD that must be explored in future research.

While our knowledge of suicidal ideation is limited, we have a great deal of research on the impact of major depression on women.

Effects of Depression on the Mother's Physical Health

We know that depression has immediate and longer-term negative effects on women. Long-term physical effects of major depression in the general population have been reported. Depression is a risk factor for heart disease (Kop & Gottdiener, 2005). Depression has also been associated with an increased risk for Alzheimer's disease, dementia, and cognitive impairment in later life (Rosenberg et al., 2010; Saczynski et al., 2010; Wilson et al., 2010).

We know that symptoms of PPD impair a woman's ability to administer self-care, disrupting her ability to respond to her physical needs and those of her infant (Bernstein et al., 2008). It is not uncommon for women to suffer from more than one mood or anxiety disorder at a time. When this happens, co-occurring mood and anxiety disorders often contribute to impairing maternal self-care and, in turn, a woman's ability to care for her infant (Henshaw, 2007; Murray, Cooper, Creswell, Schofield, & Sack, 2007; Paris et al., 2009). For example, eating disorders have been reported in the postpartum period (Franko et al., 2001; Heron et al., 2004). When an eating disorder occurs at the same time as PPD, a woman and her baby are at higher risk of nutritional deficiency (Nunes et al., 2010). When more than one disorder occurs, such as obsessive compulsive disorder (OCD), panic disorder, or posttraumatic stress disorder (PTSD), women experience even higher risks of impaired sleep, eating difficulties, lack of concentration, and thought regulation (Abramowitz et al., 2002; Bowen, Stewart, & Baetz, & Muhajarine, 2009). Substance abuse can co-occur with PPD, impairing a woman's ability to meet basic needs for herself or her infant, and increasing risk of accidents, risk-taking behavior, and suicide attempts (Ross & Dennis, 2009).

Effects of Maternal Depression on Children

We know that PPD has negative effects on infants, children, and adolescents (Campbell et al., 2007; Goodman & Tully, 2009; Mora et al., 2009; Murray et al., 2011). Many studies have demonstrated that young children exposed to maternal depression exhibit behavior problems (Brennan et al., 2000; Campbell et al., 2007, 2009; Kim-Cohen, Moffitt, Taylor, Pawlby, & Caspi, 2005). An association between maternal depression and insecure attachment to the mother in infancy has been well-established in the literature (Murray et al., 2011). Exposure to maternal depression before the age of 2 has been associated with increased risk for depression in offspring up to and through adolescence (Halligan, Murray, Martins, & Cooper, 2007; Hay, Pawlby, Waters, & Sharp, 2008). Severity and chronicity of a mother's symptoms influence the children's symptoms. The more severe and chronic the mother's symptoms, the more symptoms the children are likely to have. The severity and chronicity of mothers' depression often co-occurs with socioeconomic risk factors and racial/ethnic minority status (Pascoe et al., 2006).

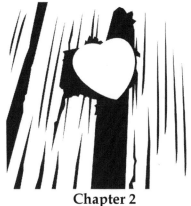

Chapter 2

Before PPD

Everything was set, I was ready to go back to work and then this just threw an entire curveball. I just wasn't prepared for just the emotions and my anxiety and it really kind of came to a head when I realized that I shouldn't be sitting in our lactation room, crying every time I pump, because that was the only place that I could let go.

—Paula

Across the board, women reported being unprepared for the PPD. With no education from prenatal care providers, when the symptoms did occur, women felt a sense of being caught off guard, stunned by the symptoms, and uncertain as to what was happening. Vicki described, "I just never had any idea of what depression was until it hit me the way it did. Everything was fine and then it was just like, Bam!"

Symptoms and Preconceptions about PPD

What I titled as the Before dimension of transformation through PPD included the mismatch between reality and expectation, lack of knowledge about symptoms, and beliefs about the world before the onset of symptoms (see Figure 1). The underlying thread, however, remained the lack of information regarding mental health in prenatal care and education. Care providers and childbirth educators failed to provide basic information on the existence of PPD altogether, much less risk factors, symptoms, or resources. This failure to provide needed information Before PPD set a precedent for what would be an ongoing and increasingly alarming trend in provider failure to address women's mental illness as the symptoms progressed. As Jamie shared, "Nobody on my birth team said anything to me about postpartum depression." Morgan said that her providers failed to give her information about PPD before the birth of her daughter. When the symptoms did occur, Morgan recalled:

It took me completely by surprise. It took me by surprise because I didn't know what it was, and why it happens to some and not others. When I was in my throes of postpartum depression, I just didn't know what was going on with me at all. I mean, no one had warned me about postpartum depression, I had no educational materials and my OB/GYN never warned me about it. I didn't understand what it was.

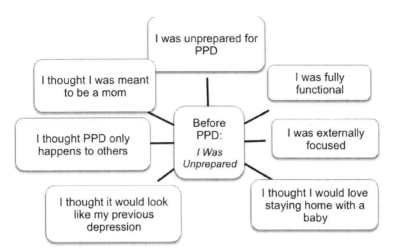

Figure 1. Representation of Symptoms Before PPD

Georgia's experience echoed a lack of preparation, such as care providers failing to discuss symptoms in prenatal care.

None of my obstetricians ever mentioned postpartum depression or anything like that in any of my prenatal visits. They had never asked me about my own history of any kind of mood or anxiety issues. They just never brought it up in any way.

The same proved true for childbirth classes. Stephanie shared, "I attended an eight-week childbirth class and PPD was never mentioned once" and Haley said, "I took a birthing class. It was never discussed other than a cursory thing."

Interestingly, women who had a history of depression or anxiety Before PPD also reported feeling unprepared for

PPD. There was a sense of confusion between what symptoms felt like Before PPD, and the actual symptoms of PPD, as Janis explained:

I did have some depressive episodes in the past so I thought I might have depression when my daughter was born. I had no idea what that would look like though. I thought it would look like my previous depression episodes of anxiety.

Vicki reflected that as well.

I didn't realize before I got PPD how many issues I actually had because my life just sort of functioned. I didn't have to have a child to worry about, and if I was OCD about something it didn't really affect anybody. So I like to say, I didn't realize how messed up I was until I actually got PPD.

For others, shameful beliefs about PPD, mental health, or women who got PPD contributed to the experience of being unprepared. Morgan explained that before she got PPD, "I thought PPD was mind over matter and I would not let myself succumb to it." Preconceptions of how women should handle PPD contributed to shame, fear, and confusion when their own symptoms developed. Preconceptions of what PPD would look like contributed to confusion and shame regarding the experience of symptoms. For example, Betsy said:

I had some very negative points of view on what postpartum depression was and I just kind of felt like, there are cases where it's really extreme, but there's a lot of people out there who are just having a hard time adjusting and maybe they didn't want the baby and like all these horrible thoughts—and now I cringe thinking, oh my God, how could I have ever thought that?

These thoughts and beliefs about the symptoms and the experience of getting through it contributed to a startling disconnect. When women became ill, they could no longer recognize who they were, as Morgan described:

I went from a highly functioning, multitasking individual with X number of years of work experience, to someone who couldn't sleep, couldn't eat, and suffered from panic attacks.

Women described picking up a mirror every day and seeing a stranger—not recognizing the stranger, not knowing what had happened, but knowing that it is something very bad. Each day, the mothers described expecting to see the mother they thought they would be, and never seeing it. These women never saw themselves function as the mothers they believed they would be Before PPD, and it crushed them.

Preconceptions about Motherhood

Mindy said, "I had this idealistic picture of the way being a parent should be . . . it was, like, way over the top." Stephanie simply stated, "I thought I was meant to be a mom." Betsy said:

I was not the mom I thought I would be, caring for a newborn, not liking it, etc. You have so many other dreams and images of what you're going to be like with a newborn, and I wasn't any of those things.

Faith's experience echoed:

I am the oldest on both sides of my parents' families, and I was always the one that babysat and took care of all the kids. I always had a kid on my hip. And so, for me, to feel the way I did about my own baby scared the hell out of me.

Skye described:

I felt very prepared for having a baby. I had been an older sister and a babysitter from the time I was little, and a preschool teacher. And so I felt like motherhood was going to be a very natural thing for me and just expected completely for it to be a good experience. I mean just hearing my child cry inconsolably, that's very triggering to hear a child. And that happens a lot with babies! And you can't always calm them down or fix it. And so it's like wow, you know, no one told me when I had a baby that I'm going to be triggered a lot.

Beatrice, who had worked with children, described the disconnect in this way.

I really had this whole philosophy of "I was going to breastfeed and cloth diaper and co-sleep and un-school." Like not even like traditional homeschool, no, I'm going to go totally rogue un-school . . . Before you had your children, you thought you would want to do those kinds of things. I mean, I was a child specialist. I worked with abused children: play therapy. What I went to grad school for is, like, family therapy, play therapy, and a child specialist. And so I really believed, "It'll be great. I'll be great with kids." I don't know why it never occurred to me before I had kids that I would be unhappy staying at home with them. It had never occurred to me that I am someone who would not be happy at home with children all day.

The repetition of *never occurred to me* in Beatrice's description underscored the lack of preparation for what PPD brought, and how it altered previously held beliefs. For a child specialist to have her own children, and then experience a completely different self, was clearly a shock. My sense of Beatrice's experience was of someone having just been hit in the head, trying to shake it off—trying to regain orientation.

This lack of recognition, combined with no prenatal education about PPD, created an overall disequilibrium. Women were stunned by what was occurring, as the symptoms took hold. In effect, when symptoms did occur, women did not recognize them as PPD, and they did not recognize themselves as they did before. Georgia told me a story that summarized the experience of Before:

When I graduated from college, the younger girls in my sorority wrote us these little books with impressions of us as the seniors. Mine said a lot of things about how confident I was, and how they all knew I was going to go on to do great things. During my PPD, I remember reading that book and thinking, "This book can't be written for me, because I don't recognize this person at all."

The process of transforming through PPD began with an ending—an ending of all that was known before. The experience of Before was shock, fear, and disorientation caused by lack of preparation before women had their babies. The result was surreal and frightening. As disturbing as these stories were, they foreshadowed a progression of symptoms that terrified women. Looking back on it now, I don't think I was prepared for what I would learn about the impact of PPD during the worst moments.

Chapter 3

I Was Shattered
(and No One Picked Up the Pieces)

I would say the process was both physically and emotionally shattering. I just felt so raw and open. I was this open wound, and that was the part of the shattering. It cracked me open in a way that everything stung like salt. I felt like I could never heal.

— Helena

Part 1: I Was Shattered

As women transformed through PPD, they described a sense of complete deconstruction. The physical and psychological symptoms of PPD, combined with their providers' failures to screen, treat, or refer them to other professionals, resulted in women being shattered. The force of PPD broke women apart. They had no point of reference, no context, no language for the physical and psychological symptoms they experienced. In the wake of being unprepared for when symptoms developed, women were confused, disoriented, and terrified of what they were experiencing. Sienna described:

> *I think it was terrifying and devastating going through postpartum. Absolutely the scariest thing I've ever gone through—and the worst thing I've ever gone through in my life.*

Betsy's description mirrored Sienna's so closely. Listen to the similarities:

> *PPD was the scariest feeling I had ever felt in my life. I didn't know what was going on. The hours ticked by and then the days, I just—it was so frightening. I felt like I was going to die.*

Physical Symptoms

Several women described PPD as a sense of falling down, collapse, crumbling, or tumbling down. The experience had directionality. For example, Dana described:

> *Within a couple weeks, I totally plummeted to the point that I was emotionally and psychologically pretty catatonic. My husband came home one day and found me sobbing, glazed-eyed on the couch. One kid was in a diaper,*

nothing else, and I don't know where the other one was.
I don't think I'd fed them hardly all day, and everything
came tumbling down.

Women also described a sense of breaking apart. Anna recounted, "I remember feeling like something cracked open, and I just literally fell to the floor sobbing." Paula described, "Basically, it leveled me emotionally, and mentally, and physically, and spiritually." Haley explained, "My whole world was split." Diana's description echoed, "It just took me to pieces and then I had to put it back together."

Pain

Recovering from birth and caring for a newborn wreaks havoc on women physically, psychologically, and emotionally, especially when they live in a culture that does not take care of its new mothers. The theme of pain or sense of physical injury and wounding was pervasive. (See Figure 2.) Anna described:

It physically felt painful. I—my heart raced and my chest
felt tight. I had a horrible lump in my throat and I phys-
ically hurt from the emotions. I just remember feeling al-
most physical pain from the depression of it all and the
anxiety.

Jamie described her pain in this way:

I remember telling my husband "I don't remember any time I wasn't in pain because the surgery hurt, the labor hurt, breastfeeding hurt, recovery hurt, and I was just like, I'm just a bag of hurt."

Loss of Appetite

The loss of appetite was another physical component of PPD for several women. Morgan said, "When I was depressed with postpartum depression, I physically could not even stand the thought of eating and I lost weight quickly. It was pretty alarming, actually."

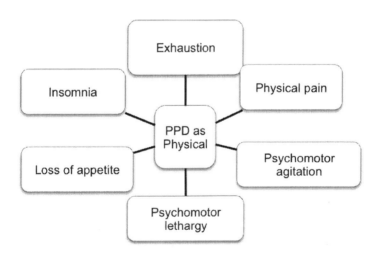

Figure 2. Representation of the Physical Components of PPD

Skye shared:

I wasn't eating very well. I would pretty much only eat things that I could just throw in the microwave and warm up. I wasn't cooking anymore. And, you know, at the time I don't think I recognized it at all as depression. I think I just felt like I was just so overwhelmed with the baby.

Insomnia

In addition to pain and loss of appetite, a significant physical component of the experience of PPD, echoed by many, was insomnia. Janis recalled her insomnia in this way:

I had several nights of just not sleeping. I just sat in the nursing rocker and had the baby. She slept and I nursed on and off, and I watched the clock. I was absolutely exhausted.

Sienna described the progression of her insomnia in this way:

It started out not being able to fall asleep, then not sleeping at all. And it went on for nine days.

Still in treatment for PPD during the time of the interview Sienna noted:

I don't have any more anxiety or depression. I just still can't sleep solid through the night. But I know one day, hopefully soon, it will come.

For those readers who may have not experienced insomnia due to a major mood or anxiety disorder, I think it is important to note that the insomnia reported here, and noted in the research literature, is that of a progression of not sleeping, graduating to not sleeping at all. When women report they were not sleeping, *they literally mean they were not sleeping.* They were awake. No dozing off, no cat naps. I often sense that the insomnia for a woman suffering from a PPD gets lost in the general understanding of symptoms.

Physical Fatigue/Agitation

There is also the experience of physical exhaustion or agitation that comes with symptoms of depression. Different than insomnia, these symptoms are physical manifestations of depression as extreme lethargy where a person has no energy to function, or their body has a sense of restlessness. In either case, these symptoms don't go away. Like insomnia and lack of appetite, being constantly fidgety, or not able to move your body out of bed, are physical symptoms that don't get better on their own. Paula describes it this way:

Really, I think the fact that, physically, the not being able to sit still was really—I felt like I always had to be doing something.

Alternatively, Vicki remembered her experience with lethargy, "I couldn't get out of bed, I couldn't shower, I couldn't function." Skye told of her experience of physical exhaustion from PPD during a move from Alaska to Colorado, when her baby was 3 months old. "I remember it being incredibly difficult to even pack. I just felt exhausted all the time." Helena's description echoed:

I was always tired. I couldn't sleep. I couldn't eat. I couldn't do my basic needs. And yet I was expected to kind of run this marathon of motherhood through this gauntlet of arrows coming at me, and boulders coming at me. I felt like I was running with sprained ankles, and gashes, and just all these things, and I could never heal, I could never catch my breath.

The Combination of Physical Symptoms

When combined, the experiences of insomnia, no appetite, psychomotor agitation/lethargy, exhaustion, and pain were described as physical collapse, or a falling down or breaking apart, with a sense of raw, ongoing physical pain. Like symptoms of any illness, they are present until the illness is treated. A person with an infection, for example, runs a fever. The fever is a symptom of the underlying infection. Until the infection is treated, the fever remains. Walking outside, taking a warm bath, drinking warm milk, having a nap, or even taking an over-the-counter medication, like Tylenol, will not fix the symptoms if the illness is severe. For women with severe PPD, like those in this book, the fever didn't ever break, until they were so sick from the infection that their lives were threatened. This was due, in a large part, to the fact that no one ever told them they might get ill, or what it might look like if they did.

Unprepared, women were shocked at the physical components of PPD. With no reference as to what was occurring or how to understand physical symptoms of PPD within normal range of postpartum physical adjustments, that shock became extreme and pervasive fear. Women were terrified by the symptoms. A similar theme was noted in the experience of the emotions and thoughts presented by the psychological symptoms of PPD.

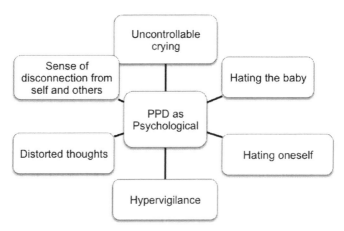

Figure 3. Representation of the Psychological Components of PPD

Psychological Symptoms

Women described that During PPD, they had emotions, thoughts, and feelings that they did not understand. Not understanding these symptoms contributed to the constant sense of terror (see Figure 3). For so many, sadness was described as uncontrollable crying. Jamie reflected, "I was crying every day with him, all day. I couldn't stop crying." Skye said, "Sometimes when the baby would cry, I would cry. I would just sit there and cry with him because I didn't know what to do." Betsy shared, "I literally could not stop crying. I remember thinking, how could I possibly not be like dying of dehydration because everything I drank just came out in tears. It was just constant." The repetition of words, metaphor, and description of not being able to stop crying clearly depicted the symptom, but also the sense of the symptom as severe, persevering, and distressing. Notice how Georgia's description begins to demonstrate a shift in description from symptoms of sadness, to symptoms of trauma.

Georgia shared, "I was definitely in triage mode after my first son was born." She described coming home from her first doctor's appointment following birth, "Like, I just sobbed, and sobbed, and sobbed, and sobbed. And of course, I didn't know at the time that that wasn't, kind of, a 'normal reaction' to that." Triage mode describes Georgia's experience of the symptoms of PPD, with the language of emergency. Similarly, Vicki recounted a social event during which she experienced unsettling and unfamiliar emotions as traumatic.

We went to dinner the night before for my husband's birthday, and I cried through the whole dinner. I cried at how I destroyed our lives. It was very traumatic, and I still remember it to a T. I can't remember anything about my son's early months, but I can remember my postpartum to a T, and it was very, very traumatic.

Turning Points

The word *traumatic* began appearing in the descriptions more frequently. This was an important finding in my analysis. Clearly, women were describing their experience of the symptoms of PPD as traumatic. But bringing in a predetermined definition of trauma before I had completed the analysis was out of bounds for the research method I used (See Appendix 1). Pressing on through analysis meant continuing to move back and forth between the text, looking for common themes, then analyzing the relationships between the common themes. This is important because it allowed the women to define their experiences, not me. The practice of getting out of the way of the data is a cornerstone of grounded theory research, the research used in this study. To that end, I intentionally set aside definitions and kept working with the stories.

For example, the split between how they thought they would be as mothers and how they saw themselves displaying emotions, was described as destructive. Having been unprepared before PPD, women were deeply distressed, expressing fear, terror, and trauma. Confusion and fear was exacerbated by feelings of ambivalence towards their infants. Women who had thought they were "going to be great mothers" were faced with feelings of anger and indifference toward their babies. For Beatrice, her experience of her own emotional state with her baby was equally shocking:

> *I was really a big believer in attachment parenting, so I carried her, like, 24/7. We co-slept. I breastfed. I cloth diapered. I was compelled to do this perfect mothering, but at the same time hating—pretty much every minute of it. I would sit and cry while I breastfed and thought, "Well, at least I can give her this," but was not enjoying it.*

Similarly, Stephanie shared:

> *It felt like I hated her a lot of the time. Like… I hated the baby. And when people would say, "Oh, she's so cute," I would nod and pretend, but I didn't really feel like that inside.*

Faith, who "had always had a baby on her hip," explained:

> *I never, in all three of my experiences, never felt like I wanted to hurt them. I just didn't want anything to do with them because I was terrified of them. I was clueless, completely clueless.*

Hypervigilance

It is important to also note that women were both aware of their symptoms and horrified by them. Mindy shared, "I thought I was a horrible mom. I couldn't understand the thoughts I was having. I really just chalked it up to being tired." Betsy described asking her husband to take the baby because, "I didn't really feel like I should be around because I thought whatever was wrong with me was contagious in some way." Helena also experienced herself as having hypervigilant thoughts:

> *The amount of hypervigilance, the amount of almost paranoia, the fear of something happening to my child was so severe, I was awake so much of the day and could not sleep and when I did, my sleep was riddled with nightmares. It was a constant, almost hopelessness that if I should let down my guard for a moment, then it's going to be over. I'm going to die, she's going to die. She's going to be kidnapped.*

Paula echoed an experience of hypervigilant thoughts concerning her baby. Her description expressed the distress experienced, and the difficulty articulating the depth of the distress:

> *I worried about everything, what the girls ate, how they were doing . . . I couldn't really articulate how I was feeling, but I knew I wasn't going to hurt—they ask like the basic questions, really trying to assess was I in any type of crisis and at that time, no, but I knew I wasn't feeling right.*

For Skye, an ongoing sense of worry and lack of feeling for her baby was devastating:

I just couldn't shake the feeling that something was going to go wrong. I felt very much disconnected from the baby. I remember kind of looking at him and just not feeling much of anything; it was almost like I was looking at someone else's baby.

I started noting that when women talked about this part of their experience, their descriptions became less cohesive. Their voices trailed off, or some stopped talking altogether for a moment. And for me, as the researcher going over this material hundreds of times, I noted in memos that I felt deeply sad every time I came on this next material. Undoubtedly, because my own suffering through PPD influenced this, and I worked to methodically follow the guidelines of research to weed out bias, and weave in what it was I was connecting with in sitting with these experiences. This was a difficult part of the research for me emotionally, and the next stories may be difficult to read. But the depths of suffering laid out below speaks volumes when you see how these women transformed after. Nothing short of a testimony to women's inherent strength, and the human spirit's ability to survive and thrive.

Hallucinations

For many, intrusive thoughts, disconnection from the baby manifested as hallucinations and dissociation. Note the language similarities between Anna's and Sandy's experiences of some of their most severe symptoms.

My eyes didn't look like me, my face; I didn't look like myself at all. I did not feel like myself. I felt like this other person had taken over my body because the thoughts I was having and the reactions I was having were just so unlike myself. There is so much not trusting yourself and not feeling like yourself and kind of feeling like the real you is kind of watching all of this take place.

Sandy's description closely resembles Anna's.

I remember staring at myself in the mirror and thinking, "That's not me in the mirror." And it didn't look like me in the mirror. When I went into the OB's office, it was like my body was in the chair, but I was watching myself from above. I totally disconnected that day. I slid downhill pretty fast that day. I wasn't myself. This is not normal. This is not me.

Karen's experience describes her most difficult moments.

I started hallucinating. I was so fearful that if I moved, I was going to die, that I couldn't move . . . it was like I had a panic attack so bad that I couldn't move. And so I got admitted to the hospital by my parents' house.

Notice the long pause in Karen's sentence where the…
is indicated. That is where Karen stopped talking in the interview. Silence. She paused for several moments before she
finished telling me that she ended up hospitalized for her
hallucinations. I was starting to realize that in many ways,
the language used in the interviews mirrored the lived experience of severe PPD symptoms: language of questioning,
repeating, pausing, slowing, losing track of the subject of
the sentence. For example, take a look at Vicki's experience:

> *I remember the first time we wanted to pick up a pizza
> and we went to jump in the car together and it was like, "I
> can't go. I can't go. No, I have to stay here with the baby.
> I just can't get in the car and go." And that was actually
> the night my postpartum started. It was the night after
> Christmas. We went to get takeout. I realized I couldn't
> go, and it was just, "My god, I can't go. I can't get in the
> car with him and go."*

Vicki repeated "can't go" six times in that passage. Something as simple as realizing she could not get in the car and
go for pizza the way she had many times before—shattered
her understanding of the world. As her PPD progressed,
Vicki's thoughts became more extreme. As she told me this,
her sentences were filled with more repetitions, broken by
pauses, and patterns of stopping and starting.

> *Constantly I would constantly just tell my husband "Oh,
> let's give him up for adoption. He's a blond hair, blue-eyed*

boy, he's... someone's going to snatch him up in a minute." And... my husband would always say to me, "Let's give it a year; let's see how you feel in a year."... So I was convinced when that year was up, we were giving him up, we were going to give him up for adoption.

To live these thoughts and feelings devastated Vicki. Vicki's words captured the end result of untreated PPD in this way:

I ended up basically suicidal. I had a lot of suicidal thoughts; driving my car into a tree, and if I wasn't going to do that, I was going to move to Florida, and my girlfriend lives there. I was going to get a job at her restaurant, and just start my life over.

Suicidal Ideation

Unfortunately for the majority of these women, suicidal ideation presented as a prominent subcategory theme. The frequency of reports of suicidal ideation was an unexpected finding. There was nothing in my research design or screening questions about suicidal ideation. I was so shocked at the prevalence of thoughts of suicide in my data, that I went back in and asked all 20 women to take an online survey. Results are presented in Table 1. Of the 20 women responding, 14 (70%) reported having intrusive thoughts of self-harm or suicidal ideation during their experience of PPD, and 15 (75%) reported experiencing PPD as life threatening.

Table 1 - Suicidal Ideation

	Number	Percent
PDD as Life Threatening		
Yes	15	75%
No	5	25%
Thoughts of Ending Life		
Yes	14	70%
No	6	30%

Knowing that the majority of women had dealt with thoughts of suicide gave credence to what I would then uncover in their stories. These descriptions were striking. For example, Beatrice said, "I really felt like dying, not like to an attempt level of suicidality, but just definitely a latent level of suicidality." Similarly, Dana reported:

> I became, I would say, mildly suicidal. I didn't actually take any steps, but I had the full prescription of my antidepressant and kind of sat there calculating, "If I take all of this, would it be enough to kill me or will it just be enough to maybe cause irreparable harm to the baby and then I'll have to live with that for the rest of my life?"

Sienna also experienced thoughts of suicide relating to overdose. In her explanation, there is a sense of accumulation as she lists medications.

Every night, I would tell my husband to take me to the hospital because I didn't want to live. I was taking my Zoloft. The doctor prescribed me at one point Ambien and Ativan, which didn't work. And I also had pain meds from my delivery, and I also had trazadone and I would want to take all of them because I wanted to sleep so bad, but I didn't want to die, so I knew, in the back of my head, I didn't want to die so I would give my husband the pills after I took them at night and say, "Hide these." And that's what we did for probably a good month.

Her words run together, almost increasing with a sense of speed—this reads as an expression of her experience. I noted that as women got more detailed about their suicidal thoughts, the details were clear, but the sentence structures diluted. For example, read Diana's description.

I went to one psychiatrist and his answer, he was very old school, was just to give me new prescriptions every week. So my medications were changing every single week. He was giving me all these, like, ones that made me totally out of it, and I was taking them and then I just had it. One night, I called my sister—she lived down the street. And I said, "That's it, I'm taking my all medicine, I'm done." And she came down, and I went into a mental hospital for, I think it was nine days. I was definitely suicidal. I don't know if I—if my sister hadn't had shown up, like, right down the street, then I probably would have taken a handful of pills, yeah for sure. But I didn't, I didn't get that far because she got there. My sister and my mom

were, like, "I don't understand. We just did it; we just got
through being a mom; you've got to just do it." And I was
like, "I'm trying to just do it." I tried "fake it until you
make it" as long as I could. And I was getting it done, but
I sure did want to die.

Did you catch it? "I sure did want to die." If I hadn't
had my interviews transcribed, I may have missed it myself. Underneath the description of events, underneath all of
the words—"I sure did want to die." The sense of wanting
death was revealed through thoughts, such as Paula saying "I did suffer from intrusive thoughts. They were pretty
horrible, most of mine involved me falling down the stairs
or getting into a car accident." There was also a deep and
pervasive desperation to end their suffering permanently.
Anna described:

My lowest moment was probably when I was in the car by
myself and I thought, very rationally, that the oncoming
MACK truck that I should turn in front of it and that
way, I wouldn't be a burden to my family, who was in
such pain watching me suffer.

Many women discussed how their thought processes
around suicide included a drive for finality. As we heard
from Dana, she had calculated how much of her medication she would need to consume to die and not still live, but
incapacitated. Importantly, women specifically noted that

they didn't so much want to die, as they wanted PPD to end. Georgia's story explains this clearly.

One night I was lying in bed, and I thought—my apartment building was seven stories high. I thought, if I go up and jump off the roof, I don't know if I'll die because I didn't know if seven stories was high enough to actually kill myself. I thought I definitely don't want to be a vegetable. If I'm going to do this, like, I need to die. I didn't see any—I didn't want to die, I just really wanted to sleep. I just wanted everything to stop. I couldn't, I just couldn't handle it anymore. So finally, that next morning, I went to my husband and said, "Like, something's wrong because I thought about throwing myself off of the building last night, and I have no idea what's going on with me."

As Georgia and others described, wanting to die was, in and of itself, a life-threatening experience of symptoms During PPD. Fortunately, there were no suicide attempts. Yet how can that be? As close as these women got to acting, with plans and access to means of completing suicide, not one attempted. For many, the symptoms of suicidal ideation became a turning point from which they were able to finally access care.

Similarly, of the 20 women in my study, 15 reported suicidal ideation, and three women who reported intrusive thoughts of harming their baby, but not one acted on those thoughts. This finding also underscored the severity of those symptoms and marked a transition from suffering to getting treated for PPD. Sandy shared:

The day I ended up getting hospitalized, I woke up that morning, and I had silent little voices in my head. I wouldn't say that I had psychosis, but I was heading towards a psychotic break. I had little voices in my head that just whisper, "Let go. Just let go because you can't do this anymore. You're tired, just let go and if you just take a pillow and . . ." Every time I walked by my daughter's room that day, it was really tempting to get a pillow. Once it started getting really overpowering, I just went into our bedroom, closed the door, curled up on the bed, called my then husband, and I was, like, "I need you to come home."

I had the overwhelming urge to actually act, and thank God, right before I knew this wasn't right. I remember rocking back and forth and saying, "I just don't want to be Andrea Yates. Just don't let me be Andrea Yates." I remember that day very, very clearly.

Women knew that something terribly negative was happening, yet due to the lack of preparation in the Before dimension, they did not know what it was. This added to the experience of extraordinary distress and contributed to the terror they experienced in the During PPD dimension. Furthermore, when women sought help for their symptoms of PPD, trusted care providers failed to acknowledge, validate, treat, or refer women to appropriate resources. The distress of symptoms was exacerbated by the stress of attempting to get help and not receiving it.

Part 2: No One Picked Up the Pieces

Nobody—my obstetrician, none of my obstetricians had ever mentioned postpartum depression or anything like that to me in any of my prenatal visits, they had never asked me about my own history of any kind of mood or anxiety issues. They never brought it up in any way.

—Georgia

For the majority, care providers failed to address PPD, even when women self-disclosed severe symptoms and asked for help. Obstetric/midwifery, general medicine, family medicine, pediatric, mental health, and childbirth professionals were sought out by women for help with symptoms of PPD to no avail (see Table 2). Women's descriptions of care provider failure included inaccurate diagnoses, prescription medication given with no explanation or follow up, referral to providers, who, in turn, failed to return calls, or were unavailable for extended periods of time, and repeated negligence to ask about symptoms. The resulting experience was an additional layer of suffering added to the physical and psychological symptoms already occurring, and reflected the nature of being unprepared.

Table 2
Provider Failure

Prenatal	Medical	Mental Health	Pediatric Provider	Labor/Postpartum Providers	Others
Childbirth Education	OB/GYN	Psychiatrist	Pediatrician	Lactation Consultant	Partners
	Medical	Therapist	Visiting Nurse	Doula	Multiple Providers
	General Practitioner	Counselor			
	Family Practitioner				
	Emergency Department Physician				

Prenatal Education

Several women shared a sense that providers failed them, even before the birth of their child. Haley shared, "I mean, I took the birthing class, it was never discussed, other than a cursory thing." Stephanie reported, "I had an eight-week childbirth class and they never mentioned it once."

OB/GYN Providers

Many women experienced provider failure from their OB/GYN. The lack of response to repeated attempts to get care was a significant component of the experience of PPD. Helena told me that after she told her doctor about her symptoms, "The OB was like, 'Oh, you just need to get out and buy a dress.'"

Diana, who experienced suicidal ideation throughout her second pregnancy and after explained:

I tried to talk to my OB about it. I was, like, "You know what? I think I'm ready to talk to somebody." And she just said, "Well, I can give you a number for someone. But they're just going to tell you that what you're experiencing is normal." And I was like, well, then screw it, I'm not going to go open my heart out to someone who's going to say, "This is normal."

Sandy also described negative experiences in accessing care for PPD with her first daughter:

I was 12 weeks postpartum with my first daughter, and made an appointment because I knew things weren't quite right. He told me, "Well, you know you're more than four weeks postpartum and your hormones should be back to normal by now and you should be fine. This isn't postpartum depression." He refused to medicate me because I was nursing.

Haley said, "If I hadn't been proactive myself, I don't know if my OB would have picked up on it because I lived with depression for a while before ever seeking out help."

Faith had PPD following the births of all three children. With her first baby, Faith said, "I think I went to three different OB/GYNs, and none of them were able to explain what was happening. So nothing. We just toughed it out." She and her husband toughed it out with baby number two as well—assuming there was nothing to be done because the doctor didn't know what to do! Having suffered twice, when she became pregnant with the third, Faith took special care in choosing a provider. She asked several sources for a referral to someone who would be able to care for her PPD. Faith explained:

I had interviewed him before. He was someone that a couple of people in a health system gave credit to for helping some women through postpartum depression. But I completely fell through with him. He did not care for me for the panic and the anxiety. I do feel like he let me down. I ended up under the care of an emergency room physician who quickly prescribed anti-anxiety, medication that my own OB had not suggested happen. I don't know what happened, and I don't know whether it was something that was meant to make me be stronger. But I certainly fell through, and it took two and a half years to heal from all of that. So—and I in turn, became addicted to anti-anxiety medications.

Despite Faith's best efforts to insure she would receive appropriate care, yet another OB/GYN failed to provide care.

Midwives

Jamie experienced a home-to-hospital transfer of care for her birth. Her birth team consisted of her midwife, an OB/GYN, labor and delivery nurses, a doula, and a midwifery apprentice. Jamie shared:

Nobody on my birth team said anything to me about postpartum depression or birth trauma when it was clear—crystal clear—from the moment my son was born that I needed mental health care. I was crying every day with him, all day. I couldn't stop crying. I was constantly upset and everybody said to me, "Well, you know, if you think you have postpartum depression, then call this number when you get home and everything." And I just remember thinking, are you looking at me? Like, what is wrong with you?

Vicki also experienced an unexpected transfer from homebirth to hospital for the birth of her baby, and shared:

My midwife was not helpful in any way. She didn't come to the house at all after what happened to me. Once I went into the hospital, I was under an OB's care, and he didn't have any clue about who I was before. My midwife called maybe twice, but she lives in the same town. She lives pretty close. She knew that I was under quite a bit of stress. She called my husband, maybe once, or maybe twice.

Having been failed to be cared for by her midwife, Vicki sought care from a family practitioner, who also failed to address her PPD. Vicki recalled:

I wouldn't send my worst enemy to him now because he didn't help—he should have said, "No, you can't leave this room until you have help." I went to him, like, three times and he was not supportive in any way. I was, like, "Something is physically wrong with me." I thought I was having heart attacks. He just said, "You need to calm down and go to sleep." And it was just so not helpful. It was really bad. I ended up in the ER three times in one week.

Similarly, in explaining the care she received for her PPD, Morgan noted the failure of her OB/GYN, and then insufficient treatment by a general practitioner:

Well, let's see, it wasn't my OB/GYN, it was my general practitioner that kind of knew what I had, but he never really referred to it as postpartum depression. He prescribed me Paxil, and when I asked him why he would put me on an antidepressant if I wasn't feeling down. He said, "Well, depression and anxiety, it seems like you have a bit of both. There's a fine line separating the two of them." He knew I was having difficulty sleeping. He knew I was on Ambien. He didn't go into any great detail of why he was prescribing me Paxil over any other antidepressant. Maybe it was successful for most of his patients that experienced something similar to me. And because I was experiencing panic attacks, he put me on Xanax, which I was on for a couple of weeks. Somehow, I survived.

Mental Health Providers

In addition to obstetric, midwifery, family and general medicine care providers, some women shared that mental health services failed to help. Janis told me:

I ended up going to—needing urgent care because I couldn't get into psychiatry for treatment. I started working with a therapist, started seeing a therapist and then was waiting to get some medication. So I was waiting to see the psychiatrist. Every single moment felt so incredibly painful and frightening. I ended up going to the emergency room for help. I felt more vulnerable than I ever have.

Beatrice shared how her experience with a psychologist resulted in her not getting the care she needed:

The professional help I did try, the lady was honestly very, very rude to me on the phone. We kept playing phone tag, and finally, when I got a hold of her, she literally said to me, "Like, what do you want?" Like, very meanly and rudely, and I was just so taken aback especially since I had training as a therapist. It was so inappropriate. I had explained to her what I was going through and she said, "Well, I'm too far for you to drive," and she didn't have anyone—any other name to give me. So I just didn't reach out for help after that.

Diana, who ended up suicidal and hospitalized, reported similar provider failure when she sought help from a psychiatrist.

I tried to go to a psychiatrist, and they told me to turn on my iPod when my baby cried, and then I went to a therapist, and she's like, "I don't know what's going on." And she said, "Do you think you're the only mother to ever experience anxiety?"

Helena also experienced provider failure from mental health professional who dismissed her asking for help with inappropriate feedback. "They said, 'Oh, it sounds like you and your husband are really struggling. Let's focus on the marriage.'"

Pediatric Care Providers

Other postpartum care providers were sought out for help, and failed to acknowledge, address, or provide care even when asked. For example, remember Sandy ended up with thoughts of harming her daughter due to lack of treatment. She had sought support from her daughter's pediatrician, and recalled:

> *I remember talking to my daughter's pediatrician. We actually begged him for a night nurse for her and he was like, "Why do you need one?" I'm like, "I'm not doing well because she needs to be fed around the clock. We're exhausted. He has to work. And I'm pumping 24/7, and we need someone." And he's like, "Well, your insurance and Medicaid won't cover it." And he refused to, and he like practically laughed at us about it. I'm, like, I need this help and you're just laughing about it?*

For Anna, who was having thoughts of driving her car into oncoming traffic, it was a visiting nurse who failed to provide much needed care:

> *Here's this visiting nurse here to help [the baby.] She goes through the checklist and she says, "Oh, are you having any postpartum depression thoughts? Oh well, clearly you're not having a problem with that." And she literally checked her box off and moved on.*

Lactation Consultants

For Betsy, problems with breastfeeding resulted in attentive care from lactation nurses and lactation consultants; however, the care provided was for breastfeeding and failed to address Betsy's PPD symptoms:

No one, even though I had been, like, to all these nurses and lactation consultants trying to breastfeed, no one had—they all just stared at my chest and my baby. Nobody actually talked to me and asked how I was doing. I remember we had this one lactation consultant who, actually, I really liked, who came in for, like, the whole day to be with us. She's like crazy-lactation-consultant-to-the-stars woman. And I haven't seen the video, but I've seen the photos, still photos from that day, and I looked so bad. There's no way anyone in their right mind could look at me and think that I was okay. Because I've seen enough women postpartum now to know, you know obviously no one looks great physically, but you know. You're tired. I know how I looked the second time around, and I'm sure I looked tired, but I also was happy and could smile and could—like my eyes didn't have that glazed over look, you know. And I remember her being really sweet and nice about—and telling me, in terms of the breastfeeding issues. And making me feel like that was okay and being very comforting. But she never asked—you know, she asked me everything about how I was feeling and his birth. Why didn't she ever just look into my eyes and say, "How are you?"

Doulas

As previously noted, part of Jamie's birth team included a birth doula. Birth doulas are trained to provide emotional support to the laboring woman during her birth, and provide resources and support for a woman in the immediate postpartum period. For Jamie, her doula was yet another source of provider failure due to not screening or acknowledging what she experienced as immediate and obvious mental distress.

> *My doula never said anything to me about it. But when I went to that therapist postpartum there was a day when I went with my son because I couldn't get a babysitter and guess who came out before me? My doula. I was about 4 months postpartum, and she was about two and she was with her baby and crying. Later I sent her an e-mail and I said, "I don't want to be nosey, but I saw you in a psychiatrist waiting room and we hugged and I hope that wasn't awkward. I didn't want to violate your boundaries. I just hope that you're okay." She said, "Oh, this is the second time I've had postpartum depression." And I thought, why didn't you share your story with me? That would have been great you know.*

Partners and Family

In addition to care providers failing to acknowledge and respond to women's symptoms, some women reported that their partners or family members failed to provide basic care despite their obvious signs of PPD. Mindy shared an experience with her husband:

> *Even though I told him I had a postpartum mood disorder, he just dismissed me, then when I started working on my photography project about PPD, he was dismissive of that until he actually heard some of the audio of women speaking about their PPD. Then I think it started bringing out fear in him. A few times he actually said, "Do I need to take the kids from you?" That was how he responded to all of this. As opposed to listening, it was all fear-based.*

Similarly, Skye described her husband's failure to address her worsening symptoms.

> *He left and went to work. Here I was, sick, with this newborn sitting next to me, and I totally felt abandoned, and overwhelmed, and sick, and it was awful. I mean, it was terrible. And I know my husband's a good man, but he was just feeling overwhelmed with the pressure of "I have to make this money for us and stuff." So I don't really blame him, but it's hard not to sometimes. It's like, really? I was totally sick. But I don't even think he was around enough to really realize how sick I was or how bad it was.*

Conclusion

The heartbreak and frustration described did not occur in isolation from the experience and demands of motherhood. The women in this study experienced debilitating physical and emotional symptoms of PPD while simultaneously engaged in caring for their newborns including breastfeeding, physical recovery from childbirth (including wound care), and returning to normal daily functions of work inside and outside of the home. In some cases women were caring for multiple children, or had additional stressors of an out-of-state move, or postpartum uterine infection, difficulty breastfeeding, or mastitis. The consequence of the multiple obstacles to treatment was a worsening of symptoms as demands to care for a newborn and return to daily functioning increased. Navigating the maze of the healthcare system and persevering through provider failure to recognize or treat symptoms created a dangerous progression of symptoms. Several women expressed a series of failures from multiple providers, contributing to an experience of hopelessness, distress, and confusion.

Provider failure, suicidal ideation, or thoughts of harming the baby were dominant features of During PPD. In addition to experiencing symptoms and struggling through the provider failure described here, women were also charged with caring for a newborn (and other children), recovering from birth, breastfeeding, returning to daily activities, and resuming work outside of the home. Diana recalled the feeling of being in a "whirlpool," while Helena described:

Part of my frustration was with trying to navigate the health care system because I was trying to reach out—I thought, maybe, these might be exit doors or ladders to get out of the maze or something. And I just kept having one door after another shut on me. It was like, who will listen to me? That's why I had to keep running this gauntlet because nobody was seeing it, only I was, and it was very lonely. There were a lot of dark hours because it seemed like every time I tried, again, another door shut in my face. I did keep trying… but a lot of women don't.

As I analyzed this data, images of the walking wounded came to mind—as if these women were hemorrhaging—in public—and no one noticed. The experience of being visibly symptomatic and yet invisible to providers was a profound feeling of complete and utter despair in flesh and form. To walk through daily life dying and being ignored by care providers, and invisible to support systems was crazy-making and cruel. There was almost a punitive sense of the experience of care provider failure—an additional layer of humiliation, indignity, and negligence. The lack of reaction from providers was an insult on top of the injury. On some level, the systemic lack of treatment created the causes for the growth of powerful resilience and determination. In other words, women got pragmatic; if their providers were not going to fix the problem, they would do it themselves.

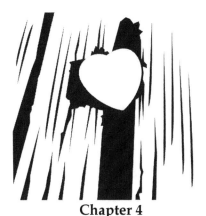

Chapter 4

Ending PPD: Getting Better

No one can do this but me. I have to figure out a way to get through this. And that's when I realized okay, you have to work. You have to figure this out. That was the moment I started getting better.

—Jamie

Given the gauntlet of symptoms and lack of information or provider care—how did women get better? I asked the question—*What were the ways you saw yourself transforming?*—to probe for specific patterns related to how women transitioned from shattered to transformed. For every woman, stopping the symptoms was a turning point in the process of transformation. As noted, disclosing to providers that they were sick didn't end the symptoms. They weren't treated or were told they had to wait nearly two months for treatment. Those who were given treatment were either given the wrong treatment, such as the wrong medication, or were treated by emergency department doctors rather than specialists. Women knew that they were receiving random, if not haphazard, prescribing of medications. They heard the condescending suggestions of buying a new dress, or turning on the iPod when the baby cried. At the intersection of the most severe suffering and recovery—women knew they were being given bad treatment, no treatment, or insulting anecdotes.

Diana told me stories of the ridiculous group activity exercises she was asked to do during her hospitalization, yet still found being admitted helpful. She shared how she would pull a particular nurse aside for advice and conversation, and just endured the sing-along music therapy. For Diana, "Inpatient was helpful in that I got a break, and I got to get away, and I got a couple good pieces of advice."

Sienna, who spent a month having her husband hide her medication every night so that she wouldn't overdose, told me how uncomfortable group exercises at outpatient treatment were for her: "We had to go every day and talk about how suicidal we were and how we were feeling that day." But then she explained that she had been so sick from her depression, it was worth it—"I was so desperately seeking a cure, seeking to get over it, I reached out to every avenue and did everything possible."

Doing Whatever it Took

Ending the symptoms meant enduring indignities and embarrassment. Still, regardless of the quality of care, women made choices that they wouldn't otherwise make, in order to have the symptoms end. Janis, who had a history of mood or anxiety disorders, had discontinued medication before she became pregnant. Following the birth of her baby, she quickly re-established her medication protocol, despite her fears about side effects. Haley, who had "lived with depression for a while before ever seeking help for it" became proactive in her care, telling her therapist that she needed specific help:

I just kept soldiering on and marching through it. It wasn't until I took the time to kind of really listen to my body and myself that I realized that I needed help. So, I called and within, I want to say, like, two days of my first phone call, I was meeting with my therapist and a couple weeks later, I was started on medication.

Haley did the work of getting better herself. She called the therapist; she waited "a couple of weeks" to get treated, which also meant enduring those weeks while still very, very ill from depression and taking care of a newborn. She then handled taking psychotropic medication for the first time in her life, while trying to understand side effects, how and when to take the medication, and waiting for them to actually work (psychotropic medication can take up to four weeks to address symptoms).

Haley's experience reminded me of someone with a debilitating migraine headache, having to call the doctor, wait two weeks for an appointment while still having the headache and taking care of a baby. Then taking the medication, and putting up with uncomfortable side effects until a month later the headache starts to subside. Can you imagine?

With no follow-up care provided after the emergency department doctor prescribed powerful anti-anxiety medication, Faith told me that she had to get treatment for dependency on anti-anxiety medication. A soft-spoken mother of three with no prior history of substance abuse, Faith's soft Southern voice described, "I would do it all over again. I would do the panic and the anxiety medication again because I don't think I'd be here today if I hadn't." Ending the symptoms of PPD, including active suicidal ideation, was essential to living. Faith knew she would have attempted suicide if she hadn't gotten herself to the emergency department. And while becoming addicted to anti-anxiety medication was a horrible side effect, Faith knew it saved her life.

Disclosing Symptoms

The heavy lifting of healing included women disclosing the gravity of their symptoms to others not knowing what the response might bring. Women did it anyway. They faced unknown outcomes of disclosing their illness and braced for the fallout—determined to do what it took to get better. Paula, who had been plagued by intrusive thoughts, told me how she had reached a turning point when she disclosed to a family member:

I knew I couldn't keep going like that. So I called a cousin of mine who is a social worker and told her, "I need to be seen right away. I need you to help me." She was my lifeline—I finally said out loud for the first time, "I think I'm suffering from postpartum depression." As soon as I got the sentence out, I burst into tears. I knew that I was—if I didn't get help, I was going to be in a crisis at some point and I didn't want to take that chance.

Paula told me that then she asked her cousin to write down exactly what to say, "so that I would be seen right away, but so they wouldn't think that I was a danger to myself or to my children."

Jamie shared with me how she finally admitted the extent of her symptoms during a phone conversation with her therapist:

I told her, "I just can't do this anymore. I feel like I've fallen through a hole in space and time, and I feel like somewhere, there's the real me, living my old life where I don't have a baby and I'm happy and I'm confident and I'm like I used to be. I'm in this universe that's all wrong, where everything's just wrong. And I'm not supposed to be a mother and this was a big mistake. You know, my husband will meet someone else. His mother will take care of the baby. I just don't want to be here anymore. I just don't want to do this and I don't think that I'm doing my son any good."

She had this answer for me that just like zapped me: "You know, I've treated people in my practice whose parents killed themselves and you need to know that your son will never be okay. And your husband, he will never be okay. Nobody is ever going to be okay. Your son doesn't need a mother, he needs you. You are the one." When she said that, I just was suddenly like, "Oh my God, like, I have to do this work, there's no other choice." I remember crying a lot and I just told her, "Okay, I'll do the work. I'll do whatever it takes, but you have to help me because I don't know what to do."

Friends

For Beatrice, her experience of getting help hinged on a close relationship with a friend across the country. As Beatrice came to describe this friend during our interview, she began to cry—almost suddenly. The tears took her off guard, as we had been talking for nearly an hour and she hadn't been tearful. When she mentioned her friend, spontaneous tears came as she recalled how her friend saved her life.

My friend said to me, "You have postpartum depression." I was like, "Well, there's nothing I can do about it. I'm in trouble, but there's nothing I can do." My friend was on a message board with someone in Miami, near me. She e-mailed her and said, "Please, help my friend. Please help her." And when that woman reached out to me... that was the beginning of getting better.

Pediatrians

While pediatricians had failed to recognize, screen, or treat PPD, for two women, their baby's pediatrician served as a lifeline. Betsy described:

I remember at my son's, I think, two-week appointment and I still, to this day, I credit her with saving me. She was so amazing. I remember she finished the appointment and she just turned to me and said, "How are you doing, Mom?" And it was the first time someone had asked me that. She said it so matter-of-factly. I was, like, okay, I need to tell somebody. That was the first time I voiced it, but I remember saying very clearly, "I think I have postpartum depression," to anyone.

Mindy received a lifeline from her daughter's pediatrician, and recounted:

When I would communicate to people how I was feeling, I was reinforced with the same things that I was initially thinking: "Oh, you're just tired . . . You need sleep." Postpartum depression was not in the forefront of my mind (or anyone else's for that matter) until I spoke to my daughter's pediatrician. I had been in to the office a few times, and this doctor saw something in me that I wasn't seeing in myself. A floodgate opened because she shared with me everything I'd been feeling, and I pushed it away. I thought I was a horrible mom. I couldn't understand the thoughts I was having. To have someone say those things out loud, and in a way that I didn't feel ashamed, was so empowering.

For Mindy, accessing complementary and alternative medicine (CAM) was a key component to her getting better. Again, Mindy sought out this care herself. Finally, getting better for Mindy also involved getting out of the house, and getting behind a camera.

I sought out acupuncture and my acupuncturist also does some therapy with it and she had experience dealing with women who had postpartum depression. I was extremely, extremely anemic. We did blood work. We talked St. John's wort. We talked antidepressants.

After I started getting treatment, I started recognizing when I had to get out of the house. I was a stay-at-home mom and all these thoughts and stuff were—a lot of the things were fear based. So I never wanted to leave the house. I never wanted to leave the kids. I had all sorts of fears. When I finally started getting treatment, and kind of had a little bit more clear thinking, I recognized the fact that I needed to get out and do something. When my son was born, I picked up a camera just to kind of keep my creative flow going, and even while I was going through this, I'd bring out my camera because if I would get really anxious or really depressed, or angry, or anything when Lucy was around, I decided to take photos.

Mindy explained to me that the experience of getting behind the lens provided a sense of cover for her symptoms while serving her desire to attend to and care for her children. Many of the mothers I spoke with struggled with the perception that their babies and children would suffer if they saw their affect. In other words, women were greatly concerned that their visual presentation of symptoms would negatively affect their babies. This concern was mediated for Mindy by using a camera. The physical lens of a camera made Mindy feel she was simultaneously shielding her children from seeing her hurting, while providing her a vehicle to express her awe-inspiring love as a mother. Using a camera might be a novel intervention for women suffering from PPD to be explored in future research.

Support Groups

Not surprisingly, many women described the role of support groups as a critical component of getting better. It is important to reiterate that while the support group was a community that helped healing, it took individual initiative to find the group, attend the group, and keep going to the group. In the middle of a crisis, women used extraordinary strength to get support. Support groups don't just appear in your living room—it takes work to find them and physically go to the meetings while juggling infant care, breastfeeding, and the physical symptoms of an illness that include extreme exhaustion. Still, they did it. Anna reflected:

> *I really felt the switch flip when I started talk therapy and medication, and within probably, two or three weeks of that, I started in our postpartum support group. That was very powerful. I just let myself be very open with women who I had never met before. I distinctly remember crying pretty much through the entire meeting. But freeing myself to be so open with strangers about something that I couldn't clearly articulate to even my closest friends or family was a big breakthrough for me. It was a blessing to have a group of people who had been through the same thing and who were describing the same things—you could swear they were reading your mind!*

Combined Methods of Recovery

Karen explained how a combination of support systems, medication, spirituality, and therapy worked in concert to help her.

> *So the first thing was the level of support that my family was able to give me. Second, I'm Catholic, so I believe in God and I believe that He gave me a gift in that [my daughter] has nothing wrong with her . . . And so, all of those things together, and my husband is really sup-*

portive. He has been nothing but supportive. And I took medication. The other big piece is that taking medication, which is, I think, the accepting help too.

Women reflected on an overwhelming sense of gratitude to the specific individual or groups who facilitated getting symptoms addressed. Women explained that finally having their suffering acknowledged was a turning point in their recovery and transformation, and many referred to this experience as a lifeline. Lifelines were in the form of resources not previously tapped. Friends, relatives, therapists, pediatricians, and support groups.

Tom Cruise

Several women mentioned anger as a motivator following an episode of *The Oprah Winfrey Show*, during which celebrity Tom Cruise made the statement that depression does not really exist. This was particularly significant for Morgan, as she explained.

Tom Cruise's rant, "There's no such thing as a chemical imbalance" opened my eyes, and I said to myself, "Wait a second, this guy doesn't know what he's talking about." And he represents, I think, most of the general population who've never experienced depression of any form. So the anger ignited within me, and I said to myself, "Well, wait a second, apparently I'm NOT the only one who doesn't know anything about it." So I decided to do something about it. The timing couldn't have been better because it was his rant that lit a fire within me. At that time, I had already started reading about what I was experiencing and why. And I said, "Well that's the most ridiculous thing I've ever heard, and if the greater majority of people out there think that way, then we're in a load of trouble." And it was a few weeks later, in July, that I decided to write a book.

Morgan's decision to write a book is an example of the transformational process. Getting better was both an end of the symptoms and a shifted worldview toward new possibilities. A critical component of the shift to recovery and beyond was the experience of being seen, heard, and accepted. The range of this experience was broad, but the underlying theme was becoming visible, finally having someone acknowledge that they had PPD resulted in a release of potential life changes never considered prior to PPD.

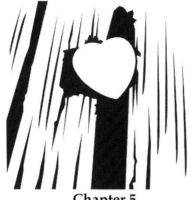

Chapter 5

After PPD:
I Was a Different Person

My experience with PPD has changed me. I call it a meta-morphosis. It's like I came out of it as a butterfly. It's made such a positive difference in terms of my attitude at work, and the attitude other people have of me at work. And this I can say for a fact because people are now telling me that they're seeing sides of me they've never seen before.

—Morgan

The fourth and final question asked of all 20 women was: *In what ways do you experience this transformation currently?* From a general outlook to specific observations, women described a process of transformation by explaining the ways they saw themselves changed by PPD, from then to now. I was struck by how clearly women knew their answers. There was no hesitation in their speech, no searching for words, no pauses. Here, the energy of the interviews developed momentum and women cited examples of how they experienced themselves as transformed with excitement and clarity. As Diana described, "So it's definitely transformed my view of the world, and my view of my life, and my view that I own my life; my life doesn't own me." A sense of clarity and wisdom about the world began to emerge. As Dana described:

> *In a more broad sense, my overall attitude and outlook on life is just a lot more positive. When things go wrong, I can generally laugh about it now, or be humorously sarcastic about it as opposed to, oh this is more evidence that the sky is falling, a "Chicken Little" kind of thing. I was just more willing to explore that kind of thinking and come out on the other side of exploring that, feeling positive and encouraged. So yeah, I think there was definitely a big shift just in my overall approach to small details and broader concepts of how you live life.*

Part 1: Transformed Sense of Self

A significant component of the paradigm shift described in After PPD was observed in changed beliefs, behaviors, and attitudes regarding self-care. Anna described new behaviors and values regarding increased self-awareness:

I feel like my experience with postpartum depression and recovering from postpartum depression really illustrated the importance of self-awareness. I think that the most marked part of transformation for me is that I feel like I work harder to be attuned to what I need and kind of checking in with myself to know how I'm feeling and what I need. Whether it's to recharge myself, or to have a physical outlet of exercise or sleep, or an emotional need for connecting with someone, or being able to vent or communicate how I'm feeling about something. I don't know that I allowed myself the time and space to do those things before that experience.

Self-Care

For some, changes in self-care involved changing how they communicated to others and eliminating negative self-talk. In our interview, Paula mentioned several times that she took a "long, hard look" at her negative self-talk postpartum, making a conscience effort to focus on positive aspects of herself After PPD. Jamie also described that After PPD she changed her self-talk. "I've learned to talk to myself the way I would want my son spoken to—with kindness. I've become a lot kinder to myself because I've figured out that self-kindness is the only way out of those dark places."

Several women discussed developing a transformed sense of self-kindness After PPD. Sandy used similar language describing that:

Postpartum depression really taught me how to take care of myself and be kind to myself. I always enjoyed doing things that made me happy, but now it's like okay, I have to do this. This is part of what I have to do to survive.

Going through postpartum created a lot of positive behaviors that I have incorporated into life now and I'm actually grateful for it. So it's a huge growth process, but for me it was really looking at myself and trying to figure out who I had become, who I wanted to be, and how much time I was willing to take for myself in the whole motherhood process.

Women put themselves first, taking their own needs more seriously than before, such as Haley saying, "I've learned to listen to myself a lot more, be a little more 'selfish' about what I need. Where before, it was more outward, making sure everyone else had what they needed." Janis said, "My prioritizing myself. I'm allowing myself to do that. It's something I have to do multiple times a day, reminding myself to prioritize me." Karen reported an important realization supporting and sustaining new patterns of prioritizing herself.

I have the realization of "I deserve to exist." And so that kind of realization of, well, "I deserve to be here," also means "I deserve to have certain things." And I've given myself the space to go slow, which is hard for me also. I like to just get things done and do it. I definitely adopted the kind of, like, I call it the Scarlet O'Hara philosophy of, like, "Oh, I'll think about that tomorrow." And that has helped me get through things too.

Going slow, listening to internal cues, and prioritizing one's needs and value distinguished the description of self-care for women reflected in the text. Transformed self-care behaviors were incorporated into daily life and accompanied by a new sense of confidence, living authentically, and being honest and open about PPD and motherhood.

Confidence

Out of 20 interviews, 17 women used the phrase, "If I can live through that, I can live through anything"—an emblematic statement of the realization of self-determination and strength in the face of extreme challenge. Women explained a sense of confidence, a sense of hard-won wisdom. Betsy said:

I felt like I had been through the worst at the beginning and lived to tell the tale so, you know, no matter what I faced from then on, I then had the tools to handle it because I had done the work and gotten through that, that initial hell.

Sienna shared, "So it feels like I've been to hell and back, you know. I can take on people. I mean, I'm just not scared of things that I used to be scared of." In strikingly similar language, Faith explained, "It's almost like I want to say,

'Don't mess with me, I have been through hell and back again, and I will knock you down just to protect this person.'" Mindy explained, "So, through this experience, I'm actually becoming a much stronger woman in my own life, and I'm continuing to move forward in that way." Haley shared the change in confidence After PPD as compared to Before PPD in this way:

I have more confidence in myself and my ability to make decisions. I'm okay. It's definitely helped me become more confident and more self-aware of who I am and what I need. I trust myself where before I wasn't. I was always doubting myself. So I'm proud of myself and, you know, saying I'm confident in who I am, for the most part, is huge.

Diana also reported new sense of pride After PPD:

Because I just feel so empowered and so strong as a person for coming through PPD. I just know that if I can get through that, and feel the way I feel now, I can do anything. I feel like superwoman most of the time.

Women also reported awareness of the increased strength and confidence emerging After PPD in their willingness to try new activities, new communication styles at work, in relationships, and approaching new relationships. Sandy reported, "I'm much more willing to go out and just explore, and live I guess, and actually, you know do things instead of just, like, I don't know if I should and I'm not as intimidated anymore." Willingness to explore and take risks was experienced as a transformed sense of self-confidence by Paula as well.

I approached someone that I admired her writing, and I knew she was a local writer to me, and I said, "Would you like to come out for coffee?" And now she and I are part of this collaboration where we're bringing storytelling experience to our city, and that would have never happened before because I would have been too afraid to be bold and to take risks.

Sienna noted her willingness to try yoga as a sign of increased confidence in this way:

And also, like trying new things, doing—I got really into yoga and Bikram. And I started that about two months ago. I started it because one I thought it would be good for mind and body. I never would have even tried or thought about doing yoga in a hot room, but it was kind of like, "Go big or go home!" I felt empowered to do it. I needed to sweat out all these bad feelings and center myself.

Sienna went on to express that her behavior at work had changed, and that her overall appreciation for life had been transformed:

I've become more empowered in all areas of my life. Things I was once afraid of, I'm not as afraid now. I'm more asser-

tive at work, a little bit. I mean, I've always kind of been passive aggressive. Now I'm not, you know, aggressive in any means, but I'm just more confident because I know that I got through that.

Reflections on the development of new strengths included new capacity for caring for themselves, and for others. Integrating honest, authentic perceptions of the difficulties of motherhood co-occurred with the experience of being less judgmental, more compassionate, and more confident to try new things and establish new relationships.

Authenticity

The ways women saw themselves transforming included increased authenticity, honesty regarding PPD, and a sense of being real about the difficulty of motherhood. Betsy offered, "It's almost like the whole experience caused me to look inward and reevaluate in a lot of ways." Georgia described living more authentically in this way:

It's almost like the postpartum depression was a gift because it gave, like, a cover under which I could go and seek help. I was, little did I know, I was seeking help for something that I had been dealing with all of my adult life for sure, and probably a good stretch of my entire life. In addition to my own healing, and finding just what I really feel like is just a better, more authentic way to live my life. I also, what the experience also gave me is, like, I don't need the cover anymore.

For Sienna, being honest and open about her experience of PPD created a transformed sense of empowerment:

I'm very open about it. I don't think I had a choice, really. I think mine was so severe that there was no hiding it. I want to spread awareness about it. I think a lot of people think that postpartum depression is equal to postpartum psychosis in that the mother kills her babies or does something, you know, kills herself. I think people get it confused. I've been open about it on Facebook, even to my over 500 friends through past college friends and everything, because I want to spread awareness, and I want to help any other mom that's going through it. I feel like I can just be truthful with people and be honest with people and I'm not really as worried about what they think.

Similarly, Sandy experienced a transformed sense of comfort with being honest with others in this way:

I'm brutally honest. I don't mince words about how I feel about something. That said, I do try to be tactful about it, but I'm like, "No, I'm not comfortable with this, so no, I'm not going to do it and it's okay that I don't want to do it."

For Paula, being honest with others in ways she hadn't been before presented through an event at work. Paula described the event in this way:

My coworker's spouse took her child's life. She was suffering from postpartum psychosis. You know it's not often that you have a team meeting and they talk about what had happened because it was in the news and he's like, "Do you have any questions?" And I just started crying in front of the entire team and I said, "This is why this is important to me. This is why it's upsetting to me personally."

We're just a small team of four, and one woman had a daughter, and she never went through it and neither did her daughter, so she really just wanted to understand. So I just really talked about this is what it's like, explained all the different mood disorders, here's my struggles, this is what I did to get better. Then with the coworker with the spouse, the same thing. I just really said, "I feel for her because here's someone in our own midst that had he'd known that I'd suffered and I blog now and I'm telling my story and gosh, I wish I knew because there are so many resources I could have given him and given to his wife." It also made me realize what a great team I had because really, the team came in support of my coworker—and my boss was really understanding.

Honesty about Motherhood

Increased authenticity was also experienced as an awareness of needing honesty regarding the demands of motherhood. One of my favorite statements came from Diana, who said, "I don't know why we won't tell each other it sucks, man." This awareness was echoed by many. Mindy described her desire to be more authentic regarding PPD and motherhood in this way:

I mean, I put so much stress on myself to try and be this picture-perfect mom, and I've realized through this experience, and through all these things, that I just need to be who I am and if I am happy with who I am, and comfortable, and confident that's going to be the most important thing for my kids. Not whether or not I'm the craftiest mom, and I'm going to hand sew all their clothes, hand knit everything, and be this incredible baker and cook. I mean, I literally had this idealistic picture.

New, realistic interpretations of motherhood replaced previously held unrealistic standards of perfection. A component of transformation involved increased authenticity regarding being a "good mom," as Karen explained:

I've realized what I kind of need as a person, and that realization of okay, these are some of the pieces of what I need to be a good mom. Things like, I need to work. I need to go outside of raising my daughter. I tried staying home for a while afterwards because it was so intense. So realizing that and being okay with that, I think, was hard for me because of that, kind of, well, my mom stayed at home with me and my sisters, and so I think there was a lot of guilt related to that too.

Paula also discussed the negative impact of adhering to powerful social constructs regarding motherhood:

I had to be supermom and I put these incredibly impossible expectations and unrealistic expectations on myself, and I would just beat myself up. It felt like I could not escape this. You felt like everywhere you turned, you saw this, like, gorgeous mom holding a newborn, with her hair perfect instead of having bags under her eyes, and a burp cloth, and wearing, like, yesterday's—you know, maybe she's still in her pajamas or yoga pants, and maybe, maybe she got a shower. It's, like, come on! That's really what it should look like.

Similarly, Georgia recognized her own new and powerful constructs of motherhood After PPD:

I love my kids, and I actively chose to be a mother. But they're not the be-all-and-the-end-all of my life. They enrich my life, and I love being their mother, and I love watching them grow up. But they're not like my purpose. Of course, that's just a very, very personal thing. But I do think, I think it's important that more and more of us manifest that. Like, "I love my kids, but sometimes I fucking hate being a mother." Like, let's be honest. I am equally as worthy of being factored into the equation. I don't, I don't sacrifice myself on the altar of my children.

Postpartum depression had made women aware of how they were holding unrealistic beliefs about motherhood. In its devastating impact, PPD gave women no choice but to be "imperfect"—to face the reality of perfect motherhood as anything but reality. Women were thankful they got to let that go, and they weren't looking back. The good mother myth died During PPD. Anna's experience suggested a welcoming of the lesson learned through increased honesty regarding the difficulty of motherhood and PPD:

> *I often say that one of the gifts of motherhood, and certainly of postpartum depression, for me ended up being that I let go of some of the very strict standards that I held myself to. I no longer feel like I have to compete with—not necessarily that anyone is setting me up for that feeling, but sometimes we can set ourselves up, or expectations of being the most creative, amazing, involved mom and I kind of let things go a little bit . . . I joke sometimes that the title of my autobiography will be,* No, I Don't Iron My Sheets and Other Crimes Against Humanity.

Clearly, the confidence women were reporting involved realistic views of motherhood, of themselves as mothers, and increased self-acceptance. Haley offered:

> *Do I make my own baby food? Do I do disposable diapers or cloth diapers? All those stupid little choices that don't really make a difference in your relationship with your child were really overwhelming for me. I always thought there was something wrong with me because I didn't en-*

joy the demands of an infant. I just—I mean, I loved my daughters. I would stare at them for hours. I loved the way they smelled. I loved the way they could fall asleep on my chest. I loved all that. But I hate the baby stage. I hate it! I don't ever want to do it again, and I'm okay with that. People look at me like I have ten heads when I say it because moms aren't supposed to say stuff like that, I guess. There isn't a discussion around having those. So you start really thinking that there's something majorly wrong with you if you don't completely lose your identity as an individual and devote everything to your child at all cost.

The knowledge of having been through PPD informed women that compassion for self, self-care, and honesty were crucial components to sustaining transformation, and new aspects of themselves that they admired. New beliefs and attitudes about motherhood were created, and old patterns were accepted. Georgia reflected that:

I still have my Type A temperament. I'll never get rid of that. But perfectionism? Fuck it. Maybe that's just me, maybe that's just motherhood. But I just don't have time or energy for that anymore. And that is such a huge gift because that's no way to live your life.

Living a life...women were telling me about living. Living a life that had been threatened by postpartum depression. The drive for life, and a commitment to living that life authentically, realistically, and fully grew from living through the worst thing that had ever happened to them. Within the new confidence and honesty, women also reported phenomenal changes in compassion for others.

Compassionate and Less Judgmental

Remarkably, every woman talked about an increased compassion or empathy for others that they didn't have prior to PPD. From the same question, *How do you experience this transformation currently?*—all 20 women discussed increased compassion. They frequently used the variations of the word give, given, and giving in describing how PPD had given them compassion. Mindy said, "Going through this experience has now allowed me to relate to other people that have gone through it. It has given me compassion and empathy."

Several told me how they transformed After PPD in being less judgmental, particularly toward other mothers. Diana said:

> *Oh, I'm definitely less judgmental. Like I—everyone— before you have kids, you're like, "Oh my God, when I'm a mom, I'll never do that." And then you have kids, and you're like, "Oh my God, anything that it takes, I will do." As I get older and I see things, and I come through the things that I've come through in life, I think I've become much more open-minded to things, and like I'm like, "Okay, you do that. I don't really agree, but that's fine with me."*

Jamie described being less judgmental in this way:

I really feel like I became, like, a much more compassionate person, and way, way less judgmental. Like a good example of that is there was a mom in the group who formula-fed and she told us, "You know what, I don't like breastfeeding. I can breastfeed, but I don't want to do it. I don't like it. So this is what I'm doing." And, you know, I found myself being totally fine with that. Before, I would have really been judge-y toward her, but now I was just, like, "You go, girl. You do whatever you got to do."

Not only did women see themselves as less judgmental and more compassionate, but they saw this change in caring for others as a gift. Here the language of suffering became the language of gratitude for having suffered and a deep understanding of the suffering of others. Vicki explained:

I'd like to say if PPD gave me anything, it was definitely an understanding of depression. I look around now at people, and I just have a whole different view: "This person must be suffering from depression." Or I think of people in jail, and how their lives have been destroyed, and how many of them must be suffering from mental disorders or depression, and just couldn't get help for it.

Janis described the ways she experienced increased compassion at work:

I'm a social worker and it's given me much greater empathy. I have greater empathy about the resources that my clients don't have and yet they have survived from the same thing. When I feel I am really struggling, I think of my clients and think of what they've gone through and survived. They had it worse, and they still survived and are moving on.

Faith noted that others were aware of her empathy in this way:

Everyone talks about my empathy level, and what I've been through to cause me to have such an empathic nature. And I do believe that. I think I was an empathic person before just naturally, but I definitely think that my experiences with PPD have made me more empathetic.

Karen described seeing herself as more compassionate and less judgmental after PPD:

But I'm realizing that I don't really know what it's like to live in anybody else's shoes, or walk down anybody else's path, except mine. I'm a big advocate now of, "do what you need to do." You know? Like, use the tools that you need because we're lucky enough to live in a society where we have access to those tools including meds and whatever else you need. So we should be able to use them then and not feel like guilty about it. So I think that change was huge.

Women also described experiencing themselves as having more compassionate attitudes towards those suffering from mental illness following their own experience with PPD. Sienna reflected on this dimension through her knowledge of her grandmother's mental illness:

It's made me a lot more compassionate to what other people are going through, especially mental illness. I have a whole new understanding for all kinds of mental illness, but especially depression. I'm more compassionate towards anybody's plight, towards any illness, cancer. I have more compassion in me for other people, and I want to help other people in any way that I can, but especially moms because that's exactly what I went through. I have a greater understanding of mental illness and like my grandmother who was schizophrenic, you know, I never really quite understood either and now I just, you know, it breaks my heart that she never really got to live a normal life.

Finally, Betsy noted both the change in views toward mental health in this way:

It was certainly never an experience that I would wish on anybody and I was very relieved not to have it the second time around, but I will say that it totally did change me as a person and make me appreciate, you know, I think whole field of mental health a lot more. I mean, my viewpoints on mental health changed, I'll tell you that. You know, it's so embarrassing, but, like, I remember—I had had a couple of miscarriages and it really made me feel like I needed to treat pregnancy like it was this holy miraculous thing. But, you know, then I was there, right there, being exactly in the place that I thought I would never be. And you know, that's really humbling.

Betsy's description of the humbling shift in a compassionate attitude toward others suffering from mental illness was followed by her discussion of the increased confidence developed through PPD.

Women's experiences After PPD included powerful indicators of change. (See Figure 4.)

Part 2: Transformed Relationships

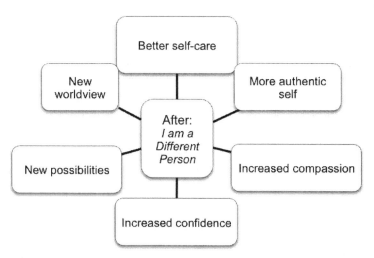

Figure 4. Representation of Components of Transformed Sense of Self

[PPD] does help you kind of break down your assumptions about people, and it is the great leveler. Women I never would have thought of becoming close friends with in my life before postpartum. And now they're a very interwoven part of my life.

—Anna

Partners

Relationships were significant parts of the ways women saw themselves transformed After PPD. Not surprisingly, women described significant changes in their relationships with their partners. Anna told me that her relationship with her husband became stronger After PPD. She explained:

So while there were some very difficult times, it really only served to strengthen our marriage and our partnership. I don't know if that would have happened if we hadn't gone through that. I think it ultimately brought us closer together.

Jamie talked about her husband witnessing her pain in PPD as a deepening:

Through it all, he supported, and he witnessed me in my pain, and in my struggle, and you know he was always there. He never doubted me for a minute. I would tell him, "I'm not supposed to be a mom. This was a big mistake.

This was a big mistake." And he was always so confident in me and he would always say, "No, no, you're good. You'll get it." And he was right. And I think, if anything, it deepened our relationship, you know, just going through such a hard time together.

Jamie went on to describe going through PPD as a couple in this way:

It was like being in a war together or being in a foxhole together. You're really bonded on a deeper level. He and I are much kinder to each other. We're much gentler with each other. We didn't fight very much before, but we haven't had a fight since my son was born. So I think we're just very, like, careful and gentle with each other, having been through PPD.

Haley explained that PPD "made our relationship stronger, the fact that he would support me and be with me through everything. I don't take that for granted at all."

For others, the transformation of relationships with partners After PPD was divorce. Beatrice discussed her ex-husband:

We went to therapy for about a year and a half, until I said, "No, I'm done." I could see myself changing during that process, and then completely changing after we separated. In terms of it being transformative, when I think of that, I think, like, absolutely it was!

Mindy also experienced a separation from her partner After PPD, and explained her view of the separation as a positive change in this way:

> *I'm moving forward. I continue to take steps forward in my life. I've separated from my husband and I don't look at that as a bad thing because right now, I'm working on finding who I am, and recognizing that I can't be in any kind of relationship unless I'm happy with me.*

Sandy described that the dissolution of her marriage involved custody of her children being placed with her ex-husband. Her reflection underscored the range of change in relationships following PPD:

> *I look back at it because everything has changed. I'm divorced now. And he has custody of the children. I'm still involved as much as I can be. We Skype every week. Ultimately, what led to our divorce was that he had addiction issues, and now I look back on my postpartum experiences, and I can't help but wonder if it was really me, or if it was the fact that he was struggling with addiction and then that weighed on our marriage.*

Now in a new relationship, Sandy shared:

> *I was on the phone with my mom and I made a comment about something that my boyfriend had done in the kitchen and she said, "Well, is he sitting right there with you?" I was like, "Yeah." And she said, "Wow, that's just huge*

because with your ex, you would have never talked about him while he was sitting there." She said, *"You know, I'm really, really happy for you because you are really just truly just being yourself now, and you're with someone who's comfortable with you being you, and you're comfortable with you being you around him, and that's just huge for you."*

Family of Origin

The perception of change by her mother affirmed Sandy's change in relationship as a positive. Changes in relationships with mothers and members of families of origin were also characterized as transformed by several women. For example, Betsy discussed a change in her relationship to her mother. When she wrote her book following PPD, she included in her writing that she had never felt close to her mother, and that the impact of the lack of connection During PPD was negative. From this experience, Betsy shared:

I think it improved my relationship with my mom, which is sort of an upside to it. And that didn't happen until much later when she read my book and she called me in tears and she was like, "Oh my God, I had no idea that you were going through that. I feel like I failed you because I didn't recognize it." And I didn't feel that way at all.

Paula engaged in new behaviors with her family, describing, "I really started taking the very scary step of interacting differently with my family, my family of origin, so my parents and my sister. Really being able to say, use my feeling words." For Janis, her unique experience as an identical twin became, central component of her experience of transformed relationships After PPD. In describing her relationship with her twin sister, Janis shared:

> *We're very similar. We both do the same field of work, and we went to college together. We have a lot of similarities at home. In many ways it's more intimate than my relationship with my husband and my relationship with my parents. I don't have any other siblings, so I don't know how the relationship is with a non-twin. But I experienced postpartum depression and she didn't. That was difficult because even though really going through my hardest time, she couldn't understand. So that has been a big transformation in my relationships. Over the years, something about my postpartum depression just changed the relationship and it allowed me an appreciation of each other in a better, different way.*

Friendships

Changes in friendships were also reported by many women. Betsy experienced an evolution in her relationship with her mother, while simultaneously experiencing the ending of a relationship with a lifelong best friend.

> *I don't think I even tried to talk to her about it because I felt like there was no way in hell she'd understand. I just*

couldn't. I don't think I could go there with her, and I think that was the first step down. Our closeness really dissipated after that. At this point, I consider her a casual friend and that is crazy, considering I talked to her more than I talked to my parents. Here was my best friend, who was supposed to know me better than anyone, and even she didn't want to hear it.

While Betsy experienced the loss of an important friendship held Before PPD, other women reported gaining new friendships After PPD. For example, Haley's account reflected, "I have forged new relationships, new friendships that I didn't have before." Similarly, Anna forged new friendships through her experience with PPD and noted the importance of those friendships in this way: "Women I never would have thought of becoming close friends with in my life before postpartum. And now they're a very interwoven part of my life."

Part 3: Transformed Self in the World

One of the most significant ways women saw themselves changed by PPD was in their considering of new possibilities for themselves in the world. Not only did women consider new possibilities: (a) new career, (b) returning to school, (c) professional or vocational change, (d) writing or creativity, and (d) volunteer advocacy—they pursued these possibilities and achieved them. For example, six of the twenty women returned to school, four women published their first book, five women started blogs, and one woman began a career as a professional photographer. See Table 3 for further details.

New Career

Remarkably, 100% reported changing career or professional paths in some manner, and attributed their experience of PPD to that change. For example, Beatrice said:

It changed my entire professional path. I decided to go back to psychotherapy as a postpartum depression specialist. I had left the field for 10 years and part of the reason why is because I went through postpartum depression. It definitely was the impetus to think, "I can do this. I think I can go back and be a therapist again."

Georgia, who had been a professional journalist, further reflected on an increased sense of gratitude for her professional transformation in how she experiences herself in the world:

Part of my transformation was totally changing my career. I left behind a career in journalism that I loved. I am actually in the course of becoming a clinical social worker, and doing the work that I do now as a therapist and that I've done in the recent past as a researcher. I think in some ways transformation is going to be happening for the rest of my life. Oh my God, I am really so thankful for it every day.

Table 3 - New Professions or Vocations.

Different Profession or Vocation	20	100%
Returned to school	6	30%
Training not related to PPD	4	20%
Training related to PPD	2	10%
Published blog	5	25%
Volunteered in PPD-Related Organizations	16	80%
Volunteered in Non-Related Organization	4	20%

Returning to School

Diana's transformation of herself in the world also involved deciding to return to professional school.

An ad came on TV for this school saying, "We have a new dental hygiene program." And I was like, "All right, well, I'll call!" I was scared to death, to death, but I was like, "I can do this, I have to do this. Like, I have to." I mean, I went back to school! I remember when I was scared to leave the living room, and here I am. I'm back at school. I have a 4.0. I'm class president. School has been the best experience for me. It's been amazing.

Professional/Vocational Changes

After her experience with PPD, Helena started a career as a postpartum doula, and eventually returned to school for licensure as a mental-health counselor specializing in working with women who have experienced PPD.

It was a very conscious effort of—it was part of my treat-
ment plan that I was making for myself, to help other peo-
ple, to become a doula, to become a mover and a shaker
in the birth community. That was a very conscious part
of my healing. It still is. It still drives who I am. I still
literally feel, sitting in the chair of the therapist now, like
moms who are struggling, how important it is to just bear
witness to their struggles, to let them know "you're not
alone," to let them know, "I'm not walking your shoes,
but I've walked that path with you, and you're not alone."

Jamie, a tech industry professional, is returning to graduate school to become a mental health professional. She
shared:

I work in the tech industry. I test software for a living.
I've always had a desire to change my career path to work
in mental health in some capacity. Before my son was
born, I wondered why I haven't gone back to school yet.
Since I've taken this journey through PPD, I realized if
I had entered the mental health profession before I went
through all of this, I would not have nearly as much to
give to people.

Skye expressed a sense of transformation in her professional counseling work:

I think the big difference this time, at this point in my life,
is that I am a counselor now, who works with pregnant

and postpartum moms. I've really been able to heal myself a lot through the work I do with other moms. Seeing myself in them and realizing that, you know, it wasn't me. I do feel like the things that I've come through, they really changed me. They changed me on every level.

Janis explained that through the experience of PPD, she realized that she needed to change her position at work:

I've changed jobs. I left the position that I had been in for three years before my daughter was born. It's the position I got right out of grad school and it was the job I returned to after my maternity leave. I realized that it was not pleasing for me any longer. It was not the work I wanted to be doing. I had to make a change and leave the position to make more changes in the way I was interacting with my work, and I've been able to do that.

Writing

Seven of the 20 women expressed that some form of writing about PPD was an extension of their transformation in the world. Dana published a book regarding her experience through PPD and noted, "After I wrote my book, I did a few activities around that. It was kind of like that's how I made peace with it and I moved on." Morgan, a financial professional, also published a book and a blog about her experience through PPD, explaining that through writing.

I put everything—all my experiences, all my thoughts, everything—into what became hundreds of pages. It took me a very long time to put it in an order that made sense. I always look back at my own writing and think, "Wow, I can't believe I wrote that." The process of educating myself through books and articles, getting all my thoughts and feelings out onto paper, putting it together in a way that made sense, working with a creative team to publish it, re-reading it at times, and sharing it with other people, helped to transform me.

Paula began writing a blog after her experience of PPD and recounted:

I really, honestly, a lot of it was inspired by some of the moms that I met online, women like Ivy Shih Leung, and after reading her book it was kind of like, "Wow, I feel empowered and I want to be able to share my story when it's appropriate, and tell people my struggles." I've loved writing, and I had forgotten how much I enjoyed it, and how much I enjoyed being creative. So it took me a while to figure out how to get everything set up, then I took the plunge probably about the spring of this past year. I've been able to help people who are struggling kind of see themselves in what I'm writing.

For Betsy, PPD created a significant professional transformation into a career change from acting to writing. She described:

It provoked a whole career change for me. That was trans-formative. I was an actress before I had my son and that's all I had ever wanted to be in my life. I never intended to totally give up acting. I just really wanted to refocus myself. But then, once he was born and PPD happened—I started journaling. Once I got better, I got really angry about a lot of things, about how we're treated as women, postpartum and prenatally. And that kind of provoked me to switch gears, become a blogger, write a book, and start trying to reach out to other women who had had PPD to make sure they didn't feel as, like, alone and lost, and scared as I had.

For Vicki, writing a grant for PPD awareness in her state was part of her experience of transformation After PPD.

So I guess a long story to, like, tell you that I think that PPD helped transform how I think about what I do—that's a big piece of my transformation. I work for the state. And when I first came back to work, I started looking at what are we doing at the state level related to postpartum de-pression or anything related to that? I wrote a grant along with another woman. The grant is to implement moth-er-infant therapy groups into home visiting programs around the state. It was pretty awesome. That's another way that I helped myself get through some of that—being able to channel it into something that I knew how to do and could work towards.

*Sandy also saw writing as one of the ways she trans-
formed. She shared: Even in the psych hospital, all I wanted was to talk to another mom because I was the only mom
there! After I got better, I looked into seeing if there were
any resources for moms in my area and there weren't. So
I started a webpage, and started a support group. I think
working with other moms in the beginning gave me something to focus on. It gave me energy outside of myself. I
realized I can help these people. I can educate myself. I can
help women find the resources that they need so they don't
have to fall as far as I did.*

*I can't tell you how many times, especially [online] that
I've heard, "I am so happy that you're doing this. I'm so
happy that this community exists because I know that I
can get on anytime of day or night and not be alone." For
me, that's huge. There's this community that exists all
because I went through hell. And for me, that makes it
worth it.*

Summary

The understanding of self-care as a mechanism of de-
serving to exist was experienced through increased compassion for self and others. Understanding the suffering of
PPD extended women's ability to contextualize themselves
in their world, and in the world relative to others. Surviving

the suffering During/I Was Shattered dimension enabled a self-confidence not previously known. Old schemas of self, destroyed through the experience of PPD, gave way to new schemas of possibilities in relationships, professional, and vocational aspirations.

The momentum for this growth was generated by self-confidence and strength gained from struggling to survive through PPD. And the momentum continued the process of transformation beyond recovery, or resilience. Women reported a dimension of transformation that included existential purpose Beyond PPD. As Sandy described:

You know you hear about people who have died and seen the light, and gone toward it and, like, given up? Then they come back, and they have a second chance. So this coming back from falling so far from what's expected to be normal and falling so far from good mental health, it just makes you grateful for every day that you have. Even when the days are hard, you know, it isn't as hard as the days back then. It's not as dark.

Chapter 6

Beyond PPD: Metamorphosis

From the beginning, to where I am now, I would definitely describe it as an awakening. I don't know why it happened when it did; why I didn't have that issue with my first daughter, but with my second. I don't know if it was the time in my life, my age, where I was in my career, or just a combination of things that came along with it. But I'm very happy with the type of mother I am right now, and the type of woman I am right now.

—Haley

The data I had gathered described being unprepared Before PPD, shattered During PPD, and the specific ways women were changed After PPD. But there was more. The nature of Beyond PPD was of paradox and purpose—questioning, wonderment, and embracing growth from adversity, women sought to put wisdom to work in their world.

Paradox

Every one of the women I interviewed for this study reported that PPD was the hardest, worst, or most difficult thing they'd ever experienced—and that they had each been transformed by it in significant, positive, and meaningful ways. For many, this began with an intrapersonal questioning as to why they experienced suffering, and what the meaning of their struggling to survive was. For example, Mindy reflected:

Part of my transformation, like, okay, I went through this. It was really hard, and what can I appreciate out of it? My goal is to try and find appreciation in things that happen to me. So instead of letting them be—dwelling on them or being this horrible side, what can I pull from this and give it appreciation?

Betsy described a general questioning.

I think, about on a very spiritual level, I wondered what was happening? Was I going through some kind of rebirth, and that's why it was so traumatic?

Georgia's experience of discovering reasons for her PPD evolved from her questioning:

I'm 42 years old, how do I parse out what's a result of this experience, and the transformation that I went through, and continue to go through? For me, a healthy portion of it is the healing, the transformation that I experienced directly as a result of my PPD, and of the help that I was able to seek. Now, I don't need it anymore. I am who I am. I'm somebody who has suffered from mental illness, and I will call it that.

Georgia's gained understanding of the transformation directly resulting from her experience of PPD was echoed by many. For Skye, the questioning reflecting on how she held ideas of herself over time. She described this experience in this way:

I felt like, "Okay, why did I feel like I wasn't a good mom when my child was one, but by the time he was 4, I felt like I was a really good mom? I'm still the same person, so what is the difference there?" It has to be that this depression really changed the way I viewed myself and viewed the situation.

Women spoke of an evolving sense of meaning regarding PPD, with both clarity and wonder. Morgan, for example, shared:

I believe I was meant to experience postpartum depres-
sion. I don't know why, I just know that I came out a dif-
ferent person. I'm a survivor and proud of it. I keep telling
myself if I could survive postpartum depression, I could
survive most anything. Sure, I lost precious bonding time
with my daughter during the weeks I was sick with PPD.
But I decided to make the most of my PPD experience. I
have accepted what's happened to me—I have no regrets.

Along with an increasing understanding of their growth
and transformation Beyond PPD, women described being
very aware of the paradox of growth coming from what
had been so difficult. How women experienced transformation currently was discussed in Chapter 5. These women
described the striking difference between who they were
in the Before dimension, and who they were now. Georgia
felt one word described the nature of the Beyond dimension
and her journey leading to it in this way:

I guess the word that comes to mind for me is "astonish-
ing." And that, I think that word encompasses a lot of
what I feel about it. For me, that something or so many
good things could come from probably, one of the worst
experiences of my life. When you think about it, if I had
gone up to the top of to that building? I wouldn't be here,
I would be dead (I subsequently found out). So I think,
wow, everyone that I'm close to, all of my siblings and
subsequently, the people that they're close to, I mean, ev-
eryone is transformed. Everyone's transformed by it be-
cause they saw it, and they know (a) that it happens, and

(b) that you don't need to just like sit by and watch it happen, and not do anything about it.

The paradox of gaining from tragedy was also reported by Faith:

It's a bittersweet blessing. But I feel like it's a blessing that I'm supposed to use. It makes me feel good about myself because it makes me feel like I'm giving back. I just feel like I'm paying it forward, I guess you would say.

Sandy also described the paradoxical nature of transforming through PPD. She described:

I know you hear a lot of women say that, "I wouldn't wish it on my worst enemy" (and I wouldn't wish it my worst enemy), but I have learned to look back at the experience as a gift, as a time of tremendous growth because I honestly think that I needed it to become the person that I am today. It really did trigger a tremendous amount of growth in my life. So the way I see it, I've been given this gift. Yeah, it kind of sucks to be depressed and need to go to the psychiatric hospital, but on the other hand, it's taught me a lot about life, living, and how to take care of myself, and how to — it's given me the ability to help others to take care of them as well.

Purpose

As Sandy reflected, the ability to put her experience to work in the world in order to help others was a significant component of the Beyond dimension. Dana described, "I don't think you can have an experience that is that massive in terms of resulting in a personal paradigm shift. I don't think you can have something like that recede into the background." Writing books, blogs, grants, hosting online support groups, Twitter chats, creating photography and videography projects to increase awareness, volunteering to facilitate support groups, reaching out to co-workers suffering with PPD, joining PPD organizations, helping other mothers, and volunteering to participate in this study were all ways women engaged in putting their wisdom to work for the benefit of others. As Sandy, now a highly successful PPD advocate with a large community, explained:

> But there's this community that exists, all because I went through hell. And for me that makes it worth it. If one mom needs help and I help at least one mom, then I've achieved my goal for the day. And that's a good thing.

Using the experience as a tool to help others were ways women experienced their transformation currently. Vicki shared:

> I know it kind of sounds bad, but I use it. I use my experience to relate to people. So, for example, some of my work in public health, I really care a lot about the isms

that there are in the world, so, like, racism, and sexism, and classism. And I think equality for people is so important. And I hope to, you know, not using it in a negative way, but use it in a way that this needs to stop. This lack of support for each other, from mental illness to if people can't afford something that they need, like, clothes, or food, or homes, like those things, this lack of being able to do that. That is what I want to—and I don't know a better way to say that, but use that for.

Mindy described an experience in a mother's support group during which she realized the need to use her experience for the benefit of others.

I would sit in this room and I'm like, "Is no one experiencing the same thing I am? I'm struggling here". . . everyone's, like, "Oh, but don't struggle. You might struggle, but you got to appreciate these moments because you won't have these moments for very long. Your kids will get old and then you'll regret it." And I'm, like, "I just want someone that can just say, 'Yes, this is fucking hard.'" So through this, I decided I am going to be that person. I feel that's why we have to go through these things.

Dana said:

I think every woman who has a chance to speak about the experience can help others. And for me, especially to be able to tag onto that experience, the positivity that came out of it at the end is a message that I'm happy to share, and circulate again and again. I think it's really import- ant for women and their families, really, who have expe- rienced this, or yet to experience it, to also know that as dark as it can be, that for many of us, there's a very, very light side of it that can come afterwards.

But I think either the difference between having had that experience, and then just assuming it's in the past, it's over and done with, "I'm not going to make any use of it," as opposed to every single one of us who experienced some kind of perinatal mental health challenge using that as motivation to try to make things better for the next group of women who are approaching that time in their life.

It's a lost opportunity if you don't do that, if you don't use that kind of situation to help others. I mean, at least to help yourself, to be able to see it for what it is, and really spend some time thinking about it, and how has it changed me as a person; that's great, and that's important, that I almost feel like it's an obligation. We're never given a sit- uation that we truly can't handle, even if at the moment, it feels that way. And that once you scale your biggest barrier, everything else in comparison is easier. And that's generally been my attitude over these last six years. Like, as miserable as it is for each of us to go through this, if we don't do anything to write about it, or talk about it, or reach out to other women, we're just kind of failing on a fundamental requirement of womanhood, almost. But for those people who have been blessed enough to have made some sort of transition, or had the ability to gain some insight, then to me that's the next obvious step, to turn it around and try to do, make some good out of it.

Helena, now a licensed psychotherapist working with women who suffer from perinatal and postpartum mood and anxiety disorders, described how she uses her own experience of PPD as a guide from which she guides others to healing:

This past year, I've been, at times, just trying to sit in the fire when it comes. Sit with the darkness and the scariness, and say, and try to say, "Okay, what is this informing me? Does it mean my life is up in arms, and it's a really big sign that I need to do a course correction," as opposed to just avoiding that feeling. Encouraging my clients in the same way toward trying to turn towards it as a sign, as a beacon for, "Okay, you're out of whack in something, and your life has a—there's something that's a mineral deficiency, so to speak, and let's figure out whether it is, so that we can improve your health again."

I think I will be transforming for a lifetime because it is one of those formative events that makes like a tree growing out of a boulder. You know, you have to—the roots are still in the cracks, and yet they're stabilizing you at the same time. And you're growing, you might, your trunk might bend, but you grow into a mentor, and then you grow up straight. So I do feel like I'm growing towards the light. I've corrected the balance, per se, even though you're always making adjustments. But my roots are in those cracks. That's what forms my entire orientation to what I do.

For Sienna, her awareness to use her experience to help others evolved from an experience at church:

The first time I went back to church, I was probably six weeks postpartum and still in the depths of it, and I had heard his message and his message was listen, if you have struggled with something or are struggling with something, don't let your struggles be in vain. It is, like, you need to reach out and help people. And there's nobody that can help other people unless they've gone through the exact same situation. And his example was rape, like, there's nobody that can help somebody that's been raped as well as another person who's been raped. Or somebody who's experienced a psychiatric illness, you know, especially like—I took it as God was speaking through him as a message to me that I need to use this experience, this devastating experience, to help other people, other moms that may be suffering.

Mindy described an awareness of her transformation through putting her experience to work in a photography project based on PPD:

It wasn't until I did that project where I was able to I think fully positively transform in my life, and move forward, because I realized, at that point, I didn't have to be stuck in these feelings, that that was part of my life, part of my pregnancy, part of my childbirth experience, but it didn't have to define me as a person . . . [Inaudible] when I could laugh about it and share it and cry about it. It allowed me to move. Also, it made me aware that this was such an important topic for all women. What I went through, what these women went through, none of us want anyone else to experience this alone. If we can stop people from experiencing it, I think, hands down, all of us would do anything we could to stop any woman from having this experience.

Georgia left a successful career as a journalist to become a licensed clinical social worker following her experience with PPD. She also now volunteers as a support group leader and advocate. She noted that she was aware of her continuing to transform in this way:

Every mom that I meet transforms me a little bit more as I learn about their experiences, and how similar, but different, what we call "PPD" or postpartum depression, how different it can be. Interacting with these moms reinforces, for me, my own transformation. It, like, manifests, it, like, reflects it back to me. And so, therefore, makes it all the more real, and the more solid, solidifying it or, I don't know, I'm having this visualization of myself being, like, I was saying kind of always in transformation, so maybe, not totally, like, whole. And each mom that I meet, like, adds another piece to me that is this post-postpartum person.

Faith explained that she is aware of the ways her transformation has extended into her current life, 13 years After PPD in similar ways:

I think through sharing with other people, I do. Because if I speak or write about my experiences, it's like I gain new insight as to how I was able to transform the way I have or how I continue to transform from the experiences.

Perception

Many women described experiencing meaningful coincidences and events regarding their connection to others. The nature of this component of the dimension of Beyond PPD was one of new or unique extrasensory perception not previously experienced. Women did not report finding these occurrences alarming, distressing, or remarkable, but a part of their awareness of ways they had experienced transformation. Mindy, for example, shared her encounter with a coincidence regarding the work on her photo project about PPD. She had enrolled in a photography class following her PPD, and went to discuss topics for a final project with her professor. She shared:

And then, it was funny, and that might be why that photo project came up at the same time because I believe that things aren't really coincidental, things come into our life for a reason. I said when I tapped on that classroom, and I'm, like, postpartum depression. I'm, like, "Where in the hell did that come from? Why did that topic come to mind?" But it did, right at that moment.

Mindy's experience of sudden suggestion, created a new perception of both the import of her transformation, and the possibility of purposing wisdom gained through suffering through her creativity. The experience of developed wisdom through increased perception for many came through their relationships with their babies. Although more subtle, women spoke of the paradox of having extraordinary bonds with children and also having struggled so greatly with PPD during the early stages of motherhood. Betsy explained her sense of the connection with her son in this way:

But there's—I don't know, this feeling of, "We were in this battle together, and we both have these war wounds, and we share that common bond." Whereas, like, when I had Lucy, it was, you know, just pure joy, and fun, and wonderful, and that's great too. It's just different.

Realization of differences in one's ability to bond, and the quality of the bond was a perception women developed through the suffering of PPD. For Jamie, this came in the form of a different kind of bond with her son than she had anticipated prior to PPD. Jamie described the word intentionality and its relationship to her son in this way:

> *I think for me, the key part of it is this idea of intentionality. So I thought that when I had a baby that I would, you know I would love him right away and that everything would just come naturally, including birthing, and it didn't. And, you know, I think one thing that was part of this whole transformative feeling that my postpartum depression gave me was that I've come to believe that there are times in our life where we love somebody because we just do, and we just fall in love with them, or we fall in love with the situation or something like that. And there are times when we really have to be intentional and say I am going to work really hard to make love grow here. And I've found that doing that produces a love that is no less genuine than the kind that just comes, sort of generates on its own. And that it feels stronger to me because my bond with my son feels very strong to me because I had to work to get it. I had to intentionally, like, try to love him.*

Several components of beyond perception emerged from Jamie's experience. Jamie confronted the loss of assumptions held in the Before/I Was Unprepared dimension regarding her birth and motherhood. Jamie realized that loving a child took work, and intention to "make love grow here." The wisdom gained beyond that realization was that the value of love that is worked on, nurtured, and intentionally purposed, was no less than the preconceived ideal of love held Before PPD. Moreover, the strength of the bond with her son resulted as a consequence of the work she put into creating it. In this way, the experience of struggling through PPD generated a bond with her son stronger than what she had imagined Before PPD, encountered During, or experienced in the After dimensions of transformation through PPD.

Dana also described a sense of connection with her son that was beyond what she had with her other children, due to their experiencing the struggle to survive PPD together. She offered:

But the other thing that was interesting is I felt at the time of Joseph's birth, and to continue to feel that I have a different bond with him than with my other kids, which of course, I could never admit to them. But because he and I went through that together, and survived the pregnancy despite my wishes otherwise in the beginning.

A lot of people will think it's just a thing inside of you that has nothing to do with it. But I really came to feel like that's where the partnership was. That it wasn't just me deciding to change my mind, and it wasn't just him having the world to survive. But it was something together.

The partnership of survival Dana described was a dimension of the transformation through PPD that extended the experience beyond recovery, or the ending of her symptoms. She was aware of the changed quality of the connection to her son.

Other observations of extended or enhanced perceptual capacities were described as awareness of the impact
of sharing one's story with a group of people. Georgia described such an experience during a training course following her PPD.

There was a day, and it was probably three or so weeks into
that eight-week course where I totally broke down, and in
the room with these nine strangers and our group lead-
er. But I couldn't keep it together; we were going around
the room, talking about bonding with my children, and I
just totally fell apart. And it was a scary moment for me
because I just remember thinking, like, they're going to
reject me.

Like people were drawn to me after that meeting—but I
also remember noticing, like, other people talking to peo-
ple, not to me. But there was more interaction among the
women. And from that point on, I felt like there was—
and when I talked about it since with them because I have
gotten to know a lot of them really well, and they kind of
felt the same thing, like something changed that day. By
sharing what I did, I allowed the other people in the room
to just, to be more real about the experience that they were
having.

Georgia's perception of the change in the interaction
between individuals signified a shift in her perceptual capacities surfacing from, and beyond, her experience of PPD.

The sense of increased empathic perception and skill was echoed by Skye. A counselor, Skye noted that:

So I do feel like the things that I've come through, they really changed me. They changed me on every level to where I can work with other women and I can sense a lot of times what they're going through and how they're feeling.

Karen also described a sense of transformation among those, with whom she shares her experience:

I will talk about it with anybody because, maybe, somewhere along the line, somebody will share it with somebody else, and it'll get to somebody else, and eventually, there will be some better laws, or I don't know, or better support, or another way to look at life. I don't know exactly what it is. But I feel like that is a huge piece of what I want to help support.

Karen's willingness to share her story as an extension of her growth was echoed by stories and narratives of other women. The ways women described experiencing transformation in their current life included examples of transformed narratives and stories symbolic of the journey.

For some, the narrative of their lives following PPD had changed in ways they described as transformational. Anna's story of the pearl earrings, described in a previous chapter, where she stopped wearing the pearl earrings she had worn every day after she came through her postpartum experience, is an example of this. When Anna stopped wearing those earrings every day, her friends and family saw it as a visible expression of her transformation. The story, the telling of it, and retelling of it, was an extension of her experience Beyond recovery. Her narrative of no longer wearing them, and not feeling badly about it, signified profound change in her life story. The story of the pearl earrings became a part of the story of her transformation.

The concept of story was mentioned by Georgia as well. For Georgia, the experience of her story Beyond PPD created an awareness of the need for narratives in all aspects of human interaction. Georgia reflected:

You know how in pretty much every culture you know, we have, we have fables, and we have stories that we pass down, and that cultures, that parents tell children and grandparents tell grandkids. And there's a reason why human beings need to do that. Like, it tells us something about ourselves, and I think that that's what I . . . I think that's what I experience. Like having conversations like this, speaking out to whomever asks me about my experience or individually with the work that I do with the women that I help is to kind of, is to, like, keep this story alive, as painful as it was.

Georgia went on to explain that her awareness of the need for her story extended beyond the experience of the pain ending and provided a link to a higher purpose and life meaning. She shared:

172

The story is all that I have now of the experience that I had, like the memories and however the memories have kind of come together into a story, that's all I have. And so I think that's why I need to keep myself kind of immersed in it, to remind myself, this is why you are where you are, and doing what you're doing.

Sharing stories of symbolic narratives was a component of the description of transforming Beyond PPD. For several women, these stories were shared at the end of our interview, or after the interview had ended, in member checking. After reviewing the transcript for member checking, Diana e-mailed the following message:

Thank you for listening to my story! It was quite a struggle, but I won! :) Oh, I was going to mention that the song, Viva LaVida, *by Coldplay came out during my suffering and I related to the lyrics of that so much.*

One minute, I held the key
Next, the walls were closed on me
And I discovered that my castles stand
Upon pillars of salt and pillars of sand
It was the wicked and wild wind
Blew down the doors to let me in
Shattered windows and the sound of drums
People couldn't believe what I'd become
I hear Jerusalem bells are ringing
Roman Cavalry choirs are singing

Be my mirror, my sword, and shield
My missionaries in a foreign field.

For Diana, the lyrics made meaning of her experience beyond her own narrative. They reflected her experience of paradox, purpose, and extended her perception of the experience into poetic verse.

Similarly, at the end of our interview, Jamie shared a tremendously significant experience for her regarding her awareness, perception, and sense of transformation by sharing this story. A year after Jamie's PPD, she went to a medium. On her way out of her session, the woman told her to check her phone. Jamie walked to her car, and as instructed, looked at her phone. She recognized the Rumi affirmation feed. The quote for the day was as follows:

I have come,
To drag you out of yourself
And take you into my heart.
I have come
To bring out the beauty
You never knew you had
And lift you like a prayer,
To the sky.

Jamie told me, "I knew in that moment, that was the lesson."

Chapter 7

Trauma and Transformation

The lesson of PPD presented in this book has been described by women as a journey of suffering and change. In order to better understand the experience, this chapter reflects on how a theory of PPD as traumatic and transformational fits, or doesn't fit, within established schools of thought on PPD. Is this really about evolution? Or is the traumatic impact of PPD and a woman's ability to grow as a result an adaptive response to social risk? Current research acknowledges that PPD co-occurs with confounding factors. The wealth of literature examining risk factors has demonstrated clearly that PPD does not occur in isolation, but rather in "conjunction with a complex interplay of sociodemographic, biophysical, psychosocial, and behavioral factors" (Jesse & Swanson, 2007, p. 378). Previous history of mental health problems, maternal age, obstetric problems, unplanned pregnancy, lack of social support, violence in the home, and poverty have all been found to increase the risk of PPD. Health psychologist and trauma expert, Kathleen Kendall-Tackett (2010), noted that we must consider the social and environmental contexts that women come from including their families, communities, and cultures. Given all that we know about PPD and the multiple factors involved with a woman's physical, psychological, and social well-being, it isn't a huge leap to consider that PPD is an experience that impacts a woman's development.

Theories Reviewed

Development, in and of itself, implies change from one state to another. Nothing is stagnant. Certainty is uncertain. No state of being remains idle. Nor can states of development be universally experienced as solely positive, or solely negative. The extreme variations on the theme of the nature of depression in science, literature, art, psychology, and philosophy truly test our ability to see the proverbial forest from the trees. For example, theories of positive aspects of depression, such as depressive realism and evolutionary theory, have changed the paradigm of depression to include stress response.

Depressive Realism

In 1972, experimental psychologist Martin Seligman published research regarding learned helplessness in the face of extreme adversity, suggesting that depression may result from a perceived lack of control over the outcome of an uncontrollable situation—such as trauma.

Not only do we face events that we can control by our actions, but we also face many events about which we can do nothing at all. Such uncontrollable events can significantly debilitate an organism: they produce passivity in the face of trauma, inability to learn that responding is effective, and emotional stress in animals, and possibly depression in man (Seligman, 1975, p. 7050).

Shortly after the publication of Seligman's work, Alloy and Abramson (1979) further challenged conventional clinical views of depression by suggesting that, "not only do depressed individuals make realistic inferences, but that they do so to a greater extent than non-depressed individuals" (Moore & Fresco, 2007, p. 144). This theory, depressive realism, stemmed from early studies demonstrating that depressed individuals have better judgment regarding the outcome of their actions, as opposed to non-depressed individuals. In this research, it was found that non-depressed individuals experienced "an illusion of control, in which they consistently overestimated their degree of control over the outcome... Depressed individuals experienced no such bias" (Moore & Fresco, 2007, p. 145).

So did the women in this book experience depressive realism? The research itself was not inquiring as to the judgment of contingent events, but the experience of the

177

events as transformative. To date, there have been no studies regarding PPD as an adaptation of depressive realism. While women in this study described enhanced empathy, compassion, and more realistic inferences regarding their needs and potentials, depressive realism does not explain the nature of the growth as a result of the experience of depression. Future comparison between transformative PPD and the mechanisms of depressive realism may be fruitful, particularly because women who develop PPD are unique in that they are mothers traditionally given the primary role of caretaking of an infant while experiencing depression. Furthermore, for women who experience PPD as a traumatic life event, depressive realism extends the theoretical discussion, but not the practical application of how that event might produce transformative growth, or personal development. What other theories consider the potential growth associated with depression that could explain the growth described in this book? Not surprisingly, anthropology and evolutionary science have examined the role of depressive behavior in human development.

Evolutionary Theory

With its stated philosophical roots in the Greek philosophy of Hedonism (Katz, 2013; Moore, 2008), and its legacy noted in the work of Darwin (1872), Lewis (1934), and Bowlby (1980), evolutionary theories of depression propose an interpretation of the depressive symptoms as adaptations to adversity (Hagen, 2011; Hammen, 2005). According to evolutionary anthropologist, Edward Hagen (2011), depression can be explained as an adaptation to adversity because it provides benefits to the people experience it.

Evolutionary theory, for the most part, theorizes malignant sadness as psychic pain or distress as a motivator for adaptive response (Hagen, 2011; Tennants, 2002; Trevathan, 2010). From this perspective, PPD might be viewed as maladaptive sadness formed as an affect adaptation to adversity that serves to recover important connections between mother and child, or mother, child, and environment. The "malignant sadness" of PPD serves to repair something broken in the vital connection between this primary and crucial dyad.

Other evolutionary hypotheses, such as social-competition theory and social-risk theory, have proposed somewhat similar theories about the adaptive function of depression. The social-competition theory of evolution determined that depression was an emotion of submission manifested to function to note rank in dominance hierarchies (Price, Gardner, & Wilson, 2007; Price, Sloman, & Gardner, 1994). Social-risk theorists, Allens and Badcock (2003), suggested that:

Depressed states evolved to minimize risk in social interactions in which individuals perceive that the ratio of their social value to others, and their social burden on others, is at a critically low level. When this ratio reaches a point where social value and social burden are approaching equivalence, the indi-

179

vidual is in danger of exclusion from social contexts that, over the course of evolution, have been critical to fitness (p. 887).

Within social-risk theory, depression serves to reduce threat by increasing sensitivity to signals of others that may threaten them, and by "inhibiting risk-seeking (e.g., confident, acquisitive) behaviors" (Allens & Badcock, 2003, p. 887). Analytical rumination hypothesis (Andrews & Thompson, 2009) proposed that low mood and sadness are responses to social adversity, and serve to trigger psychobiological and neurological responses, which, in turn, signal the individuals to solve complex problems. A trade-off of one impairment for a more adaptive impairment results. A common analogy made by Andrews and Thompson (2009) has been that depression is like a fever in this way:

Stress response mechanisms can produce impairments when making trade-offs between different body systems to respond to a stressor. For instance, fever is metabolically expensive and causes significant impairment in multiple domains (work, sexual functioning, social relations, etc.), but these impairments are not usually the product of biological dysfunction. Rather, fever is an adaptation that evolved to coordinate aspects of the immune system in response to infection (p. 621).

From this perspective, could PPD be defined as an "evolved stress mechanism" through which a woman experiences changes in body systems that "promote rumination, the evolved function of which is to analyze the triggering problem" (Andrews & Thompson, 2009, p. 622)? While this variation of evolutionary theory may foster a future understanding of the psychobiological properties and mechanisms of PPD in order to promote problem-solving skills through rumination, this hypothesis does not explain how the symptoms themselves create the conditions for profound personal growth (Hagen, 2011).

I was about one year into my data analysis when I had exhausted theoretical literature of depressive realism and evolutionary theories. I knew that based on all of the data, I was looking at an experience of trauma. PPD, as described by the women, was traumatic.

Posttraumatic Growth

Could PPD cause psychological trauma? Can PPD itself constitute a trauma? Women are exposed to a life-threatening event: PPD. They are horrified and terrorized by intrusive thoughts, hypervigilance, insomnia, irritability, physical discomfort, negatively impacting their ability to care for self and others every single day. Moreover, the lack of sleep expands the window of suffering to night. Without proper intervention, women get no relief from symptoms, and no relief from the distress about the symptoms.

Trauma psychology has been examining the ways individuals respond to traumatic life events for decades (Figley, 1978; Horowitz, 1976). The advancements in the field of positive psychology (Linley & Joseph, 2004; Seligman & Csikszentmihalyi, 2000; Snyder & Lopez, 2002) have generated greater theoretical understanding as to the positive emotional states associated with psychological well-being. As our understanding of the responses to traumatic events has evolved, we are learning that a fundamental response often includes profound personal growth.

Tedeschi and Calhoun (2004) defined posttraumatic growth (PTG) in this way: "The term posttraumatic growth refers to positive psychological change experienced as a result of the struggle with highly challenging life circumstances" (p. 1). Expanding the definition of trauma beyond the set criteria of the APA (2000), Tedeschi and Calhoun (2004), sought to "describe sets of circumstances that represent significant challenges to the adaptive resources of the individual, and that represent significant challenges to individuals' ways of understanding the world and their place in it" (p. 1). From this theoretical perspective, the experience of PPD described in my research could be defined as a traumatic life event.

Furthermore, PTG theory extends concepts of recovery, resilience, survival, to include the nature of human beings as growth based. We don't merely recover to pre-trauma levels of functioning. We grow. Our development post-trauma has momentum. Tedeschi and Calhoun (2004) explained:

Posttraumatic growth describes the experience of individuals whose development, at least in some areas, has surpassed what was present before the struggle with crises occurred. The individual has not only survived, but has experienced changes that are viewed as important, and that go beyond what was the previous status quo. Posttraumatic growth is not simply a return to baseline—it is an experience of improvement that for some persons is deeply profound (p. 4).

Tedeschi and Calhoun (2004) determined that the term "posttraumatic growth" best captures the phenomenon for several reasons. According to the authors, the term "stress-related growth" (Tedeschi & Calhoun, 2004, p. 4), used by other growth theories emphasize the nature of the stressful event, and minimized the growth potential. Terms that suggested illusory dimensions of transformative change through traumatic life events minimize the ontological reality of transformation. Tedeschi and Calhoun (2004) explained "in contrast to the terms that emphasize the 'illusions' of people who report these changes, there do appear to be vertical transformative life changes that go beyond illusion" (p. 4).

The quality of the growth experienced by women in this research was beyond illusion of stress-related growth, demonstrated by the high number of changes of vocation and occupation. The growth described was not explained as a coping mechanism. Significantly, women did not describe thriving or flourishing regarding their perceptions of the transformation. The change experienced was not expressed in rebuilding the old self, nor was it described as changing depression. Depression created the causes for one of life's essential challenges: building a new self with information and wisdom gained through the loss of the old self.

Was This Posttraumatic Growth?

It has been reported that somewhere between 30% and 70% of survivors of traumatic events experienced positive change in some form in their lives (Linley & Joseph, 2004). While the impact of the stressor is negative, the manifestation of the suffering in relation to the stressor is not universal. As I got more clarity that the findings in my study were reflective of posttraumatic growth, a lingering question remained: did the women in my study experience posttraumatic growth?

I corresponded with the authors of the Posttraumatic Growth Inventory (PTGI), and received their permission to use the inventory to perform a posttest with my original sample (N = 20). The PTGI is a 21-item self-report inventory that measures the "extent to which individuals believe they have grown positively from the struggle with the traumatic experience" (Triplett et al., 2012, p. 401). Five subscales of the PTGI include (a) relating to others, (b) new possibilities, (c) personal strength, (d) spiritual change, and (e) appreciation of life (Tedeschi & Calhoun, 1996). Responses are 6-point Likert-type scale ranging from 0 (no change) to

Table 4 - Posttraumatic Growth Domains and Transformational Dimensions of PPD

PTG Domain	Transformational Dimensions of PPD
Domain 1 Increase appreciation for life; changed priorities **Domain 2** More intimate, meaningful relationships, increased compassion **Domain 3** Increased personal strength, "If I can handle this, I can handle just about anything." (Tedeschi & Calhoun, 2004, p.6).	**After PPD: Transformed Self** (a) Better self-care (b) A more authentic self (c) Increased compassion (d) Increased confidence: "If I can survive PPD, I can get through anything." (Morgan) (e) Transformed relationships
Domain 4 Identifying new possibilities	**After PPD: Transformed Self in the World** (a) New career (b) Returning to school (c) Professional, vocational advancement (d) Volunteer (e) Creative projects
Domain 5 Spiritual and existential change	**Beyond PPD** Perception (heightened empathy, connection to spirituality, connection to baby) Purpose (increased wisdom, sense of purpose, meaning of life)

5 (great change). Total score (0-105) represents a measurement of posttraumatic growth in the amount, degree, level, extent, and number of benefits (Tedeschi & Calhoun, 1996).

The findings in the current study resembled the domains of PTG in several ways, demonstrating a theoretical connection supporting future research regarding PPD as a trauma, and transformation as posttraumatic growth (see Table 4). From the findings studying the five domains of PTG, appreciation for life is accompanied by a "radically changed sense of priorities" (Tedeschi & Calhoun, 2004, p. 6) that includes appreciation for things formerly taken for granted. The findings in this study confirm this domain in the reports of women reprioritizing self-care behaviors After PPD.

I asked the women in my sample to complete the Posttraumatic Growth Inventory (Tedeschi & Calhoun, 1996). Each agreed, and with the full sample responding, I was able to determine whether the group, on average, had experienced posttraumatic growth. The average total score was high, 74.8. On average, the women in my sample experienced posttraumatic growth following PPD.

Changes in relationships, both losses and gains, and the report of increased compassion After PPD confirmed the second domain of model of PTG, and the report of increased strength and self-confidence by women reflected the third domain of PTG theory, the general sense of increased personal strength (Tedeschi & Calhoun, 1996, 2004). The After dimension of transformational PPD involved women's identifying and achieving new possibilities in personal, professional, creative, and vocational aspects of life, mirroring the dynamic of the fourth domain in PTG theory.

The nature of the Beyond dimension of transformational PPD presented subcategories of paradox and purpose that echo the fifth domain of PTG. Women experienced a transformation in the ways they considered their existential purpose in life, increased spirituality, and increased sense of meaning and purpose for their experience of PPD. The experience extended to women beyond recovery, beyond returning to previous levels of psychological well-being, and encompassed the development of wider aspects of self-development, connection to others, sense of purpose, and existential wonder.

Chapter 8

Professional Perspectives

Researchers have focused in on the actual experience of postpartum depression and not the recovery.
So I think it's an excellent point that you bring up.
And that's an area that needs to be researched and
certainly that would lend to posttraumatic growth.

— Cheryl Beck, personal communication

As I rounded the corner on writing this book, it occurred
to me that while I had attempted to gather a full range or
perspective, I had yet to ask other professionals for their in-
put on my findings. Why is this important? From a researcher's standpoint, it is essential to get peer review. Handing
over your findings for critique is scary, but essential to the
establishment of good research. This is the first research describing postpartum depression having the dimensions of
trauma and the potential for traumatic growth or transfor-

mation. There are no other studies (believe me, I looked). As such, I wanted to offer the readers critical insight from other experts. And as you will see, I included both agreements and disagreements. Who to choose? I charted out the prominent features of my work, and asked the experts in each of the areas if they would be so kind as to read my synopsis, and tell me what they thought. I knew I needed an expert in trauma and the perinatal period, an expert in post-traumatic growth, an expert in clinical practice, and an expert in postpartum support and advocacy.

I spoke with Cheryl Tatano Beck, DNSc, CNM, FAAN about my findings and her thoughts regarding trauma, research, and postpartum depression. I then interviewed a leader in the field of posttraumatic growth research, Dr. Jane Shakespeare-Finch, to investigate the validity of my study and gain deeper understanding of PTG theory as it relates to PPD. Next, I interviewed Karen Kleiman, MSW, LCSW—one of the leading clinicians and authors in the field of postpartum mood and anxiety disorders. Finally, I spoke with Jane Honikman, MS, the founder of Postpartum Support International (PSI), whose honesty and wisdom about the state of postpartum support sent me back to the proverbial drawing board. It was a distinct honor to speak with these experts. Collectively, they broadened my vision through critical reflection, encouragement, and brainstorming. I am equally honored to share their thoughts with you.

Cheryl Tatano Beck, DNSc, CNM, FAAN: *Everything is Data*

Dr. Cheryl Beck is a Distinguished Professor at the University of Connecticut, School of Nursing. She also has a joint appointment in the Department of Obstetrics and Gynecology at the School of Medicine. Her Bachelor of Science degree in Nursing is from Western Connecticut State University. She received her Master's degree in maternal-newborn nursing from Yale University. Cheryl is a certified nurse-midwife and also received her certificate in nurse-midwifery from Yale University. Her Doctor of Nursing Science degree is from Boston University. She is a fellow in the American Academy of Nursing. She has received numerous awards, such as the Association of Women's Health, Obstetric, and Neonatal Nursing's Distinguished Professional Service Award, Eastern Nursing Research Society's Distinguished Researcher Award, the Distinguished Alumna Award from Yale University, and the Connecticut Nurses' Association's Diamond Jubilee Award for her contribution to nursing research. She has been appointed to the President's Advisory Council of Postpartum Support International.

Over the past 30 years, Cheryl has focused on developing a research program on postpartum mood and anxiety disorders. Based on the findings from her series of qualitative studies, Cheryl developed the Postpartum Depression Screening Scale (PDSS), which is published by Western Psychological Services. She is a prolific writer who has published over 140 journal articles including such topics as phenomenology, grounded theory, narrative analysis, meta-synthesis, and qualitative secondary analysis. Cheryl is co-author, with Dr. Denise Polit, of the textbook, *Nursing Research: Generating and Assessing Evidence for Nursing Practice*. Editions of this text received the 2007, 2011, and 2013 American Journal of Nursing Book of the Year Award. Cheryl co-authored, with Dr. Jeanne Driscoll, *Postpartum Mood and Anxiety Disorders: A Clinician's Guide*, which received the 2006 American Journal of Nursing Book of the Year Award. Cheryl's latest two books include *Traumatic Childbirth* and *The Routledge International Handbook of Qualitative Nursing Research*.

During the first part of our conversation, I asked Cheryl about the relationship between PPD and trauma.

WK: *Can postpartum depression be traumatic?*

Cheryl Beck: *Well, from the research I've done and listening to countless women in interviews, I do believe that the moderate-to-severe postpartum depression certainly could be viewed by some women as traumatic, not the mild, and I don't necessarily know those women, but one's that are really struggling with the postpartum depression, so I say moderate-to-severe. If you wanted to classify as traumatic, it would be then at that far right end, going from mild-to-severe, the women who have severe postpartum depression. You know, I hadn't asked women in those studies if they perceived their depression* *as traumatic. It certainly was very difficult time for them and they struggled. I never asked them about it being perceived as traumatic like I have with the women with their birth process. But I would say some of them would have, probably not all of them would have said it was a traumatic experience if we're looking at traumatic experiences as being horrified about something, fearing for your life. So I would say some, but not all, women with postpartum depression would view it as that.*

You know, many of the women in my studies talked about their loss of self. They didn't know who they were anymore. They were really afraid they would never get their old self back again. Now, I never researched women with postpartum depression viewing it as posttraumatic growth. So I haven't talked about that, but certainly, they were very fearful that they would never be back to their old selves again, let alone be at a higher place than they were before their depression.

WK: *I'm wondering, from your perspective, is it that we just need to do more research on recovery? We've got so much data about the pathology, what would you value in looking at how women recover and what the nature of that recovery is?*

Cheryl Beck: *I think you're on an excellent point. You know I have my "Teetering on the Edge" theory (Beck, 1993). I've modified it twice because Glaser [grounded* *research methodologist] always says that everything is data, and that your grounded theory shouldn't be stagnant as new research studies are done, or if you collect more data yourself. You constantly are revising.*

So, the two revisions that I've done on that theory looked at qualitative studies that had been published since I had done my original grounded theory—which was all done with middle-class, Caucasian women. So when I looked for more qualitative studies published among other cultures to expand my theory I could ask, what parts of the theory did women from other cultures endorse? Were there some new things?

It was very interesting because the least bit of research has been done on the last phase of my Teetering on the Edge theory, the recovery phase. Really, researchers have focused in on the actual experience of postpartum depression and not the recovery. So I think it's an excellent point that you bring up; and that's an area that needs to be researched and certainly that would lend to posttraumatic growth.

The questions put forth by Cheryl as she discussed her own research inspired my ongoing wonder as to the relationship between trauma, PPD, and personal growth. When I had the pleasure of interviewing Cheryl years ago, I asked her how someone knows they are a researcher, and she told me that when you wake up in the morning wondering about your research—you are a researcher. Cheryl identifies the gap in research regarding PPD and recovery with a researcher's curiosity, and her wonder as to the fullest possible range of experience for perinatal women, including posttraumatic growth, was affirming as I approached interviewing an expert in posttraumatic growth for feedback on my research.

Jane Shakespeare-Finch, PhD: *We Need to Normalize the Experience*

Dr. Jane Shakespeare-Finch is an Associate Professor in the School of Psychology and Counselling at Queensland University of Technology, where she teaches a variety of topics including health psychology, individual differences and assessment. Jane has enjoyed supervising nearly 50 post-graduate student research projects, including the completed supervision of eight PhD candidates. Jane's primary area of research is in posttraumatic growth. Starting with emergency service personnel, Jane continues to work with paramedics and police in the promotion of positive post-trauma outcomes, and has also investigated the construction of trauma, and post-trauma adaptation and growth in various populations, including refugees, and survivors of sexual assault, cancer, and bereavement. Jane is currently Secretary of the Australasian Society for Traumatic Stress Studies, a member of the International Society for Traumatic Stress Studies, and is an international affiliate of the American Psychological Association's trauma division. Jane has published seven books, 13 book chapters, and more than 70 peer-reviewed journal articles, and is a regular presenter at national and international conferences. After sending Jane my research to review, we spoke by phone. Our conversation began with her views on the research.

WK: *What are your thoughts on the research I presented regarding PPD as a traumatic life event?*

Jane Shakespeare-Finch: One of the things that I noticed that you found, and that we have found, is this notion of increased compassion for other people. That real development of empathy and compassion toward other people, which seems to be kind of a normal thing for many people who've experienced trauma and come out the other end; to want to actually be instrumentally useful to other people.

I think one of the things about your area of research is that society tells us that having a baby is a wonderful thing. And that nurturing comes naturally, you know, like latching on for breastfeeding, it's a natural thing, but for many women, that simply is not the reality. So you then have these expectations of everything going well, the birth going well, the baby being beautiful and having all the things it's meant to have, and then happy families going home and looking after babies and moving forward, whereas in actual fact it completely, fundamentally shifts who you are as a person. And when that event doesn't work the way you expected it to, there's much self-doubt and self-blame for things not working the way that the books have told you or society has told you it will. And I see that could quite easily lead to a spiral of downward affect, etc....as one beats themselves up that they don't look like the celebrities on the TV, and they're not shedding all their kilos and looking wonderful and feeling just dynamic about being a new mom.

One of the things we may fail to do in a therapeutic setting is to draw on people's strengths, to recognize them, and reflect them back. We have to normalize the experience that people are having. We've been doing quite a lot of work with sexual assault survivors recently, and the same thing is happening there. This is devastating, yes it is, but most women who have experienced childhood sexual assault do go on to be fully functioning adults—the way in which we intervene can have a lot to do with that.

WK: *What would you see as some of the gross misunderstandings about, specifically, posttraumatic growth?*

Jane Shakespeare-Finch: *I think one of the first things that springs to mind is this argument in the literature that posttraumatic growth is illusionary; that it's the positive spin people put on things to help them cope with an experience. And that's a fundamental misunderstanding about the way in which people actually do truly transform their lives as a result of that struggle that they engage in.*

I think that's one of the fundamental problems. The other is confusion between what is growth and what is resilience, which is only just recently getting a bit of air. But when you have people who are prolific in the literature sort of saying, "No, this doesn't exist. This is some sort of artificial illusionary coping strategy," then it makes it difficult for those of us who actually sit there with people who've survived trauma to be heard.

The other difference, I think, between posttraumatic growth, and some of the other concepts like thriving, flourishing, and stress-related growth is that in Richard [Tedeschi] and Lawrence's [Calhoun] model, and you've found it in your research, is that the experience has to be one that shatters your previous assumptions about the world, about your place in the world, about the predictability and safety of the world, about good things happening to good people and bad things happening only to bad people, that kind of thing, if you can use those dichotomies. And so, I think the fact that the posttraumatic growth model is solidly embedded in cognitive theory and requires that schematic shattering in order to rebuild your sense of who you are in the world and incorporate or weave that experience into your life, makes it different to some of the other concepts.

WK: *How do you see posttraumatic growth as a component of care for clinicians?*

Jane Shakespeare-Finch: I think the posttraumatic growth model is the most comprehensive and sensible model that we have to look at positive post-trauma life changes. And there is very little recognition of the fact that, for many people, the experience that can provide the catalyst for symptoms of PTSD is the same experience that provides the catalyst for growth. And these things can and do co-occur.

A psychologist's job is to sort of disentangle psychological disorder, correctly identify a diagnosis and formulate some sort of intervention whereas, I actually think a solution-based approach to trauma research and to practice is much more beneficial for the people that you're aiming to help. And this model that Richard [Tedeschi] and Lawrence [Calhoun] came up with didn't come out of thin air. It was created over 20 years, as working clinicians, as well as academics, and seeing the real changes that were made especially in the lives of bereaved parents.

One of the things that we always need to say right up front is that people finding a positive transformation through their experiences does not, for a second, deny the very devastating experiences that they had in the first instance. And that it doesn't mean that this is one outcome as opposed to another outcome, that there are interplays of many outcomes for people. As I was saying before about having a good day, but that doesn't mean that you might not hear a piece of music or see something that reminds you of a time when you were in the depths of despair and that it's perfectly all right to allow yourself to feel those emotions. Not everything in life is wonderful and glossy, and you don't want to sell posttraumatic growth as something that can be perceived to be illusionary, because it's not.

I think having really practical ways of trying to express to people that yes, you've got research that backs up what you have found here, but these are the real ways in which people, allied health professionals and people who are surviving these experiences, can engage with themselves, with their thought process, with their emotions, with their relationships with other people, to create a new narrative that isn't laden with that, "Hang on a second, this isn't the way life is supposed to be, therefore, somehow, I have failed." And that beating up of self that happens. I think we just need to be much more honest about the human condition and speak in terms that are accessible to people.

Dr. Shakespeare-Finch offered critical review of clinical implications for posttraumatic growth interventions. What struck me in speaking with her was her acknowledgment of the human condition as both flawed and filled with possibility. Underlying all of the research we have to date regarding the pathology of PPD, lays a pragmatic, solution-based sensibility yet considered—of course, women grow through suffering. The concept of growth through PPD as viewed as a traumatic life event isn't as much new as not articulated by research and theoretical literature, such as depressive realism and evolutionary theory.

Secondly, of course, women grow through suffering. We all do. As noted, growth through adversity is well documented in philosophical, psychological, and religious literatures. Traditional science and epistemologies of science have examined growth through adversity as well. From Aristotle's eudaimonism, to Carl Roger's organismic growth theory, Maslow, Rollo May, Laszlo, positive psychology, and now posttraumatic growth have examined growth through adversity as an integral component of the human condition. What has not been made as obvious, however, is the identification of PPD as one of those adversities. We don't call PPD traumatic.

As providers and researchers, how we disentangle the seeming conflicting ontologies of growth and suffering is critical to our ability to recognize growth potential in the face of adversity for women who experience PPD. As I learned from my interview with Karen Kleiman, disentangling the language of suffering itself can be problematic.

Karen Kleiman, MSW, LCSW: *Is it a Big T or a little t?*

Karen Kleiman, MSW, LCSW, is well-known as an international expert on postpartum depression and anxiety, and advocate for perinatal women and their families. Her work has been featured online and within the mental health community for three decades. In 1988, Karen founded The Postpartum Stress Center, a premier treatment and training facility for prenatal and postpartum depression and anxiety disorders, where she treats individuals and couples. More recently, she founded The Postpartum Stress & Family Wellness Center in New Jersey. Karen is featured as an expert on PsychologyToday.com as a "Best Voice in Psychology," as author of her blog, *This Isn't What I Expected: Notes on Healing Postpartum Depression.*

In addition to her clinical work at The Postpartum Stress Center, she created and instructs a professional training course for clinicians who have an interest in specializing in the treatment of postpartum distress. Karen is the author of several top selling books on postpartum depression. Her first book, *This Isn't What I Expected: Overcoming Postpartum Depression* (2nd Ed., 2013), co-authored with Valerie Davis Raskin, forged new territory in the self-help book market on postpartum depression. Frequently listed as the bestselling postpartum book on Amazon.com, Karen's book has proven to be an essential resource for women and their families. Her subsequent books on postpartum depression, *The Postpartum Husband: Practical Solutions for Living with Postpartum Depression* (2001) and *What Am I Thinking? Having a Baby After Postpartum Depression* (2005), continue to contribute significantly to the self-help market for families dealing with postpartum depression. She co-authored, *Dropping the Baby and Other Scary Thoughts: Breaking the Cycle of Unwanted Thoughts in Motherhood* (2011) with Amy Wenzel, and her book, *Therapy and the Postpartum Woman: Notes on Healing*

Postpartum Depression for Clinicians and the Women Who Seek Their Help (2009), has been a groundbreaking resource for clinicians who treat women with postpartum mood and anxiety disorders.

I interviewed Karen specifically for her feedback as a clinician with unparalleled expertise in treating PPD. How does she view my findings within her own experience? Were there elements of care provider failure that resonated with her experience? What would she make of the theory that PPD can be experienced as a traumatic life event? What is shared here are the segments of our conversation regarding (a) care providers, (b) suicidality, and (c) PPD as trauma. Karen's insights provided invaluable feedback and beg further discussion. I explained to Karen the high level of care provider failure reported in my research. Karen described her understanding of the compartmentalization of physical and mental illness by care providers this way.

Karen Kleiman: Postpartum depression symptoms are the feelings that a woman has that are expressed as symptoms, but they are experienced as self. So we say, when somebody is sick and she goes to the doctor, and she has a sore throat, and she has swollen glands, and it hurts to swallow, and she has a fever. The doctor says, "Oh, here's a cluster of symptoms. I know what this is. And I know how to treat it." And when a woman has postpartum depression, she says to us, "I'm a bad mother. I am powerless over how I am feeling. I will always feel this way. My loved ones will abandon me." And when I, as the clinician, hear those sentences, "she thinks she's a terrible person"—I hear she has a sore throat, and she has a fever. Right? I say to women all the time that this is not about you. This is about your symptoms. These are symptoms. When you get better you will no longer feel this way.

Symptoms became a theme of our conversation. When I asked Karen about the high levels of suicidality I found in my research, she shared:

Karen Kleiman: *I think we have no idea how big it is. And what I always say is if you don't ask every single postpartum woman if she's having thoughts of suicide, you have no freaking idea. And these are women that look like you and me, and are going to their doctors, and they're asked how they're feeling, and they're saying they're fine, and they're going home thinking of ways to kill themselves. Luckily the numbers aren't as high as the symptoms are, but I think that the disparity that women are faced with, with motherhood, within the context of being a mother feeling this way, mental illness aside, mental illness alone is bad enough, but you stick a baby in there? "My baby would be way better off without me." I mean, hello. You don't have to look very far to feel that way. So I think that thoughts of suicide, I think that people are missing that all over the place. And fortunately, a lot of these women are just getting better. They're just getting better. But I think a lot of clinicians are looking at these women that look really good, and look really healthy, are* *not asking them how many glasses of wine they're having a night.*

Karen's insights as to the symptoms associated with suicidal ideation in PPD are chilling, and merit attention. As part of my ongoing research for this book, I did an informal anonymous survey regarding suicidal ideation (Appendix A). I asked two questions regarding suicidality. The first question was, *Do you consider your experience of postpartum depression (PPD) to have been life threatening?*, and received the following responses. With a total of 486 completed responses and 41.2% (n = 200) responded "Yes"; and 58.8% (n = 286) responded "No." Question two asked, *Did you experience thoughts of harming yourself or others during postpartum depression (PPD)?* With 486 completed responses, 61.1% (n = 297) responded "Yes"; while 38.9% (n = 189) responded "No."

The survey results certainly supports Karen's assertion that suicidal ideation for postpartum women is underestimated. How might the experience of suicidal ideation relate to a direct experience of trauma? If trauma involves exposure to life-threatening events, would then suicidal ideation in postpartum not therefore be by definition traumatic?

The conversation with Karen regarding PPD as trauma continued to provide thought-provoking questions as to how we unpack symptoms and understand a woman's experience of those symptoms relative to the diagnostic criteria. In asking Karen about how she perceived clients as experiencing PPD as a trauma, she shared the following:

Karen Kleiman: *It's interesting as I was thinking about this in preparation to talk to you; I was seeing that my population is really split down the middle. It feels like half the women that I see, and this is just anecdotal, obviously. Half the women that I see sort of take this what I'm going use your word "trauma" even with the little small t, and not a big T. And they take this trauma, and they carry it with them as if they continue to be burdened by it forever. And they are angry, and they are tired, and they are frustrated, and their marriage is impaired, and they literally cannot move forward or let go, which is what I see is one of my greatest challenges is to help them learn that.*

The other half, and these are just women who stay in treatment, obviously, so I'm not seeing the women that get better and leave. But the other half of the women that stay are women who are falling more into the category that you're describing, who feel that maybe something good has come out of it, maybe my marriage has strengthened, maybe awareness is more acute, maybe my ability to take care of myself has been initiated through this process. And sure, I mean, we hear things like that all the time. I wouldn't wish this on my worst enemy, but I've grown into a better person because of it. And so then we know that in terms of the trauma literature that the same two people can be in the same trauma, and one of them is paralyzed by anxiety or incapacitated by their trauma. And the other one goes on to teach about it, and write about it, and save the world because of it.

So the resilience in terms of who they are is also very relevant. I have to tell you that that's one of the things that we do in therapy is talk about sort of the characteristics that are associated with that kind of positive adaptation. You know what I mean? And when I see somebody struggling, one of the things that we do, not right away, but as she's healing, is we take, literally, a list of the characteristics. Like the ability to plan, and seek support, and find humor, and insight and all this stuff. And we go through it, and I say to her, "If you're not good at these things, let's work on these things. These are the characteristics that are associated with a better recovery and a positive adaptation of this trauma so to speak."

As a clinician, Karen integrates appreciation for a woman's ability to adapt to PPD in positive ways. Through her clinical interview and establishing therapeutic rapport, Karen encourages her clients to acknowledge characteristic strengths and weaknesses in order to facilitate and promote growth and recovery. But what of the traumatic impact of PPD? We further discussed her view of PPD as trauma "so to speak." What is meant by the word trauma to a clinician with an expertise in PPD?

Karen Kleiman: But that sort of what gets me confused. The word "trauma" actually gets me confused. That's the part that I'm not sure I can articulate. I'm not sure I see this in the same way in terms of PTSD and that. I see it as something that I can't really define yet, which I probably should have done before I talked to you. But I see it as sort of the breaking down of the soul and devastation in mind, in spirit is not the same thing to me as a trauma. It's traumatic, but in terms of the definition of a trauma, I just don't see it as PTSD. I just don't see it. Now, is it there, and I'm not seeing it or what's happening? But I don't see it in my practice. And trust me, I'm looking for it. I see this other thing. I see a loss of confidence, and I see sort of the breakdown of who I used to be, and how do I get that back, and sort of that dream that I was describing, that my insides were all over the place. So I don't see that. Clearly that's traumatic, and we're probably both saying the same thing, but the word "trauma," in its clinical sense, doesn't always apply to what I'm saying.

Part of the wonderful experience of interviewing Karen is her willingness to critically unpack ideas, while infusing her own expertise. She holds her space as an expert clinician and invites dialogue that may or may not lead to mutual agreement. I love that kind of conversation! These are the conversations that challenge us to grow: reflect on what we know, review what we want to know, and reframe our paradigm. What she offers here is an invaluable reflection for care providers, scholars, and women. Struggling with the terms and their meanings as a clinician speaks to the need to reflect on how and why we use diagnostic criteria. The manual of diagnostic criteria for psychiatry disorders used predominantly by psychology and psychiatry clinicians is the DSM-5, published by the American Psychiatric Association (APA, 2013). Based in medical science, the manual provides criteria for psychiatric disorders as evidenced in medical research. In the most recent version, trauma has been given a new and separate category of disorder: "Trauma and/or Stress Related Disorders" (APA, 2013), having been moved from anxiety disorders in past versions. According to a 2014 white paper published by the American Psychiatric Association, the symptoms defined as being in response to:

...exposure to actual or threatened death, serious injury, or sexual violation. The exposure must result from one or more of the following scenarios, in which the individual:

- directly experiences the traumatic event;

- witnesses the traumatic event in person;

- learns that the traumatic event occurred to a close family member or close friend (with the actual or threatened death being either violent or accidental); or;

- experiences first-hand repeated or extreme exposure to aversive details of the traumatic event (not through media, pictures, television, or movies unless work-related).

The disturbance, regardless of its trigger, causes clinically significant distress or impairment in the individual's social interactions, capacity to work, or other important areas of functioning. It is not the physiological result of another medical condition, medication, drugs, or alcohol. (http://www.psychiatry.org/dsm5)

From this perspective, one can understand how clinicians might struggle to align PPD with trauma. The criteria, defined by medical science, must match the condition presented by the client in order to signify the disorder noted in the manual. There are many instances of disconnect between mother and medicine. Perinatal mood or anxiety disorders (PMADs) have no distinctive diagnostic category in the DSM. A clinician working with a woman suffering from PPD must look to the general disorders in the DSM for a postpartum-onset specifier, in order to find the diagnostic code to write in her medical chart. A woman doesn't get a diagnosis of PPD—in fact, there is no such diagnosis in the DSM. A woman with the symptoms of PPD is given the diagnosis of a Major Depressive Disorder (MDD) with a postpartum-onset specifier, a slightly modified numerical code that determines how she developed MDD within 4 to 6 weeks following childbirth (APA, 2013).

Another example of disconnect in diagnostic criteria for women during the childbearing period is trauma. There is no postpartum- or perinatal-onset specifier for trauma disorders. Despite solid research identifying the experience of childbirth as traumatic for some women, there is no postpartum-onset specifier in the criteria for PTSD. She may have directly experienced the death of her infant, the invasive medical procedures done to her genitals, the loss of blood, the loss of consciousness—but none of that experience matches the list of criteria for trauma. If that woman develops symptoms of distress relative to the childbirth that impair her ability to care for herself, or her infant—what diagnosis does she receive? There is none.

The powerful messages here are that perinatal mood and anxiety disorders are separate and not equal from the "real" disorders. Perinatal mood or anxiety disorders are silos related to depression and anxiety, and have no relationship to trauma disorders. Furthermore when childbearing women experience trauma as defined by the medical establishment, there is no code to apply defining her trauma as related to childbirth. The result is an ongoing and damaging mismatch between meaning and medicine.

Jane Honikman: Simple as That

Jane Honikman is the founder of Postpartum Support International (PSI). I read *I'm Listening*, by Jane Honikman, in 2007. When I received the book, Jane had included a handwritten thank you note in the package, a gesture of manners I remember to this day. I met Jane in 2010, and consider her a friend and mentor. The first time I heard Jane speak, I got very angry. Not at her, or the content, but the fact that she was slated to speak during a lunch, and how rude it seemed to me to hear clinking of silverware while she spoke. I was there to hear what the woman who had single-handedly built PSI had to say. I learned then, that sometimes when strong women speak the truth, we can forget our manners.

I have interviewed Jane before, and have had many conversations with her over the years. Jane Honikman pulls no punches, is a pragmatic optimist, and has a mind that is constantly moving to connect people in meaningful ways. She plays the flute, prefers the phone to e-mail, and has met with her closest friends every Tuesday for breakfast for the last 30 years. Jane developed PSI in the midst of the women's liberation movement in the U.S.—and speaks about feminism from a lived experience that I personally find incredibly important and valuable. Obviously, I went into my interview with Jane totally biased. That said, I knew that she would offer me the same critical eye and authenticity I had come to admire.

When I interviewed Jane for this book, I drove to her home in Santa Barbara. I sat at her kitchen table, watching her hop around her kitchen, loading the dishwasher, and preparing lunch: heirloom tomatoes from her garden, and leftover butternut squash lasagna made by her daughter-in-law, sliced avocado, and crackers. I was used to Jane's straightforward style, and wondered what she would have to say about this theory of mine—PPD as trauma and transformation. As usual, her laser-like insight did not disappoint. In discussing the current state of PPD, I asked Jane about the prevalence rates for PPD remaining the same (or higher) since she began her advocacy work in the 1980s. She said:

> *No, the rates haven't changed and everybody wants them to be worse. And so they are. That's the other thing that I witnessed over these years. Oh good grief, it's bad enough as it is. Just leave it alone and just stay with, what are we going to do about it? We need to talk about it, and tell women to be open and honest about how you're feeling. And it's not just women; it's men too. Simple as that.*

What about the thought that women experience PPD as traumatic and can grow as a result? Jane said, "Well again, my experience early on was that the people who called me said that very same thing. They said, "It was the worst thing that ever happened to me, but I'm glad I had to go through it, and now I'm going to help others." Polite enough to direct her comments generally, she offered some wise observations of the current theoretical landscape of PPD. "Walker, we keep going around in circles, and talking as if the next person that thinks it up is the first person who's thought if it. I think we just spin. And we don't support women." Simple as that.

I drove home that afternoon wondering: Is this just reinventing the wheel? Am I just adding modifiers to the word postpartum? I knew that the women's stories of trauma and growth described something different than what has been described about PPD. Much like my interview with Dr. Shakespeare-Finch, my take-away from Jane's interview was that PPD as a trauma was not as much a discovery, as a recovery of something that has been there all along—women's ability to grow through adversity. The description of the suffering associated with PPD by medical and psychological professionals has remained consistent—that's the spinning. We recycle the same descriptions of symptoms. We circle through evidence regarding prevalence, symptoms, risk factors, and negative outcomes. We spin symptoms—not growth potential. By the time I got home, I knew I had one more transcription to review—Jane's own postpartum diary.

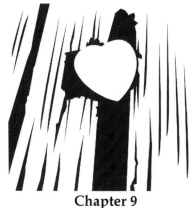

Chapter 9

PPD Grows Up: New Reflections

By the end of the drive home from Santa Barbara, it occurred to me that Jane herself had written her experience of PPD in her very first book, *Step by Step: A Guide to Organizing a Postpartum Parent Support Network in Your Community* (Honikman, 2000), and that analyzing her writing might provide final insight into the theory that PPD is traumatic and transformational. In Chapter 1: "My Postpartum Diary," Jane shared her personal diary of a difficult first pregnancy in the 1960s as an unwed young woman, her extraordinary sadness over giving her daughter up for adoption, and her experiences of postpartum depression and anxiety with her second and third baby years later. Jane's experience of PPD in 1972 echoed the women's voices from this book. Indeed, struggling to survive and transforming through that struggle was Jane's story as well. Following the birth of her son in spring of 1972, Jane remarked on how unprepared she felt, mirroring the experience of the women in this book:

I'd had an expectation that maternal instinct would wash over me and guide me through each day. It started when we came home from the security and support of the hospital. I put my baby in his cozy bed, stood beside him and thought, "Now what do I do?"

She described the symptoms of depression with falling, downward directional language similar to the women in my research, "From triumph and exhilaration of this birth, I've plunged into this morass of feeling overwhelmed and exhausted, alone, and frightened" (Honikman, 2000, p. 18). By March of 1972, Jane was struggling with breastfeeding, exhaustion, and increasing symptoms of PPD.

The baby's schedule is like a Ferris wheel in high gear, whirling and spinning. I feel like a damp washcloth being wrung out for the hundredth time as I nurse constantly. When I attended a nursing mother's group and confessed that I've been using supplemental bottles, I could feel their glares of disapproval, not to mention silent disgust. Mom came down for a few days, but couldn't or didn't want to stay. I feel incredibly alone. What am I going to do to survive this hideous existence? (Honikman, 2000, p. 18)

And as the symptoms became more severe Jane experienced care provider failure not unlike the women in this book. Jane's diary entry, from May, 1972 described:

The other day I fainted from trying to contain a pain in my chest. The doctor checked me for physical ailments, and then sent me home. He never asked how I was feeling emotionally, so I certainly didn't volunteer information about my vast sense of inadequacy, terrible mood swings, poor sleeping, lack of concentration, and anxiousness (Honikman, 2000, p. 19).

Sound familiar? Four months later, in August of 1972, Jane began to feel relief, and shared how support from other mothers was crucial to her getting better.

I've made new friends with other new mothers at a child study group through AAUW. They've helped me realize I'm not crazy or alone. It's a form of therapy, I guess. My stomach aches and headaches are not as frequent now, probably because I'm sleeping and eating better lately (p. 20).

Following a recurrence of PPD in 1974 after the birth of her daughter, Jane went Beyond PPD. In July of 1977, Jane wrote:

My vow of long ago has finally taken on a form and direction. I have a purpose now beyond being a mother and a wife, with energy coming from that unspoken force in the back of my mind. My friends and I have launched a community-based, grassroots, self-help parent support program. We got funding from a grant from AAUW. It's an idea born from our own experiences and needs. We've named it Postpartum Education for Parents, "PEP" for short, and laughed about not calling the organization "Afterbirth." The word "postpartum" is not in the public's vocabulary yet, but it is that period of time from birth through the first year of a baby's life (Honikman, 2000, p. 22).

Jane had experienced the same journey. She was unprepared, shattered by PPD twice, slowly got better, and then grew beyond better. Jane experienced growth beyond being a wife and mother, and an energy coming from an "unspoken force" that fueled new ideas, possibilities and potential, resulting in the growth of her advocacy work. For all intents and purposes, one could say that Jane experienced posttraumatic growth as a result of her PPD. And anyone who knows Jane today would tell you that she continues to grow as a result of those events. That's the message in this: growth happens With PPD, and continues to happen After PPD. We just aren't looking for it, naming it, or acknowledging it as part of the psychological construct that represents PPD. Until now. What the women in this book described, and the experts confirmed, is that there is a direct relationship between PPD and trauma. When used in relation to postpartum depression, the language of trauma expands the paradigm of postpartum depression to its fullest range. Broadening the paradigm of PPD to include the language of trauma gives the suffering its due description, as a traumatic life event.

In her brilliant book, *The Ghost in the House: Real Mothers Talk about Maternal Depression, Raising Children, and How They Cope*, Tracy Thompson described depression in this way:

...when you are surveying the wreckage of your life—and the exact cause of the devastation at some point ceases to be relevant—the question you must confront is the same one depression poses: How do I live now? The unique nature of depression is that it gets you to that question directly; no external catastrophe is required (Thompson, 2006, p. 210).

As we have heard from the women and experts in this book, postpartum depression is also such a catastrophe. It devastates all that was known to be relevant, safe, and reliable. It strips life down to the barest bones, and begs the biggest questions, such as: How do I live now? This book has shared examples of answers to those questions—as told by women themselves. Their stories are more than novel narratives of outlier moms—women who "survive" and feel a sense of cliché gratitude for the experience. This is not a collection of stories of silver linings. This book is the result of methodological analysis of the experiences of women as told by them.

The experiences of these women gives pause to consider the very nature of suffering of PPD itself, and the boundless capacity of the human spirit to grow as a result of it. Acknowledging PPD as traumatic, we also acknowledge, then, that women have reactions to it that include trauma reactions. For clinicians, this acknowledgment could identify new methods of screening and intervention that include trauma. For researchers, this acknowledgment inspires new curiosity as to cross-disciplinary scholarship between trauma psychology and perinatal psychiatry. For families, the acknowledgment that PPD is traumatic offers new vocabulary to better describe and understand PPD. For providers, perhaps the connection between trauma and PPD will serve to push through barriers of stigma regarding maternal mental illness.

How long have women waited to hear that PPD is traumatic, and that the struggle to survive it is a small miracle? How long have we known that PPD is a war for women, from which some return wounded, others, not at all? We know now that we can call it PPD war, we can call its impact traumatic, and proceed to give women who battle it the modicum of respect and care a veteran might receive. As Diana shared at the end of her interview:

One minute I held the key
Next the walls were closed on me
And I discovered that my castles stand
Upon pillars of salt and pillars of sand
It was the wicked and wild wind

Blew down the doors to let me in
Shattered windows and the sound of drums
People couldn't believe what I'd become
I hear Jerusalem bells are ringing
Roman Cavalry choirs are singing
Be my mirror, my sword and shield
My missionaries in a foreign field.

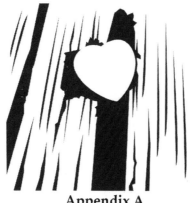

The Changing
Depression Survey

In my initial study, the four questions used were:

1. **Descriptive**: A descriptive question was employed to elicit a description of the phenomenon of transformation through postpartum depression: *How would you describe your process of transformation through PPD?*

2. **Exploratory**: An exploratory question investigated the phenomenon of transformation through PPD: *In what ways did you experience the process of transformation through postpartum depression?*

3. **Explanatory**: An explanatory question probed for patterns, processes, or categories related to the

transformation through PPD: *What were the ways you saw yourself transforming?*

4. **Emancipatory/Evolving**: An emancipatory question explored the evolving nature and processes of transformation through PPD: *How do you experience this transformation currently?*

Despite the questions being unrelated to suicide, 75% reported thoughts of self-harm, and 70% considered their experience of PPD life threatening. That was a significant finding. To explore this further following the publication of my dissertation, I conducted an informal, anonymous online survey in order to collect more data regarding suicidality During PPD and perceptions of key support figures in accessing help for PPD. I titled the survey, "Changing Depression." Recruitment was done anonymously through social media advertisement, setting an audience target to recruit women who were over the age of 20 and English speaking. I collected data via a secured, online statistical analytical service, between October 2013 and January 2014. The service maintains confidentiality and provides tracking to block repeat entries. Demographic data included age, employment, and time elapsed since the episode of PPD had occurred.

Age. The majority of respondents (n = 300; 61.7%) were between the ages 30-39; 19.1% (n = 93) were between the ages 21-29; and 15.0% (n = 73) were ages 40-49 (see Table 5).

Employment. 35.4% (n=172) of respondents reported being employed and working 1-39 hours per week. 29.8% (n=145) reported being employed and working more than 40 hours week. 28.4% (n = 138) reported not being employed and not looking for work. 4.3% (n = 21) reported not being employed and currently looking for work; and 10 respondents (2.1%) reported being disabled. No respondents (0.0%) reported being retired.

Time Elapsed Since PPD. Four hundred and eighty three of the 486 responded to this question. The majority, 56.9% (n = 275) reported it had been 0-2 years since they had experienced PPD; 25.9% (n =125) responded 2-5 years since they had experienced PPD; 12.2% (n = 59) reported 5-10 years since they had experienced PPD; and 38 (7.9%) respondents reported over 10 years since they had experienced PPD.

Table 5 - Age Range: Changing Depression Survey

Which category below includes your age?		
Answer Options	**Response Percent**	**Response Count**
17 or younger	0.0%	0
18-20	0.8%	4
21-29	19.1%	93
30-39	61.7%	300
40-49	15.0%	73
50-59	3.3%	16
60 or older	0.0%	0
	answered questions	**486**
	skipped questions	**0**

Suicidality

With a total response of 486, significant data trends emerged. I asked two questions regarding suicidality in the survey: (a) Do you consider your experience of postpartum depression (PPD) to have been life threatening, and (b) Did you experience thoughts of harming yourself or others during postpartum depression (PPD)? The question, Do you consider your experience of postpartum depression (PPD) to have been life threatening?, had a total of 486 completed responses, with 58.8% (n = 286) responding "No"; and 41.2% (n = 200) responding "Yes." Figure 5 represents these findings.

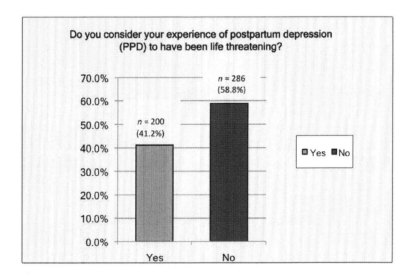

Figure 5. Changing Depression Survey: PPD as Life Threatening

226

The second question, Did you experience thoughts of harming yourself or others during postpartum depression (PPD)?, was also completed by all 486 respondents. Sixty-one percent (n= 297) responded "Yes"; while 38.9% (n =189) responded "No." Figure 6 represents those findings.

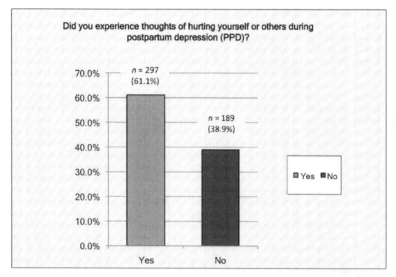

Figure 6. Changing Depression Survey: Postpartum Depression and Harming Ideation

The data here was consistent with my findings in the formal study, and more importantly, suggested the high level of suicidality in PPD may be overlooked in postpartum populations polled for research. The anonymity of the survey may have yielded higher, and quite possibly more accurate, numbers because women felt safe self-reporting thoughts of harming self or others. Moreover, given the findings in my study regarding the traumatic nature of PPD, the high levels of suicidality, and considering the experience as life-threatening, beg further research into the traumatic impact of PPD.

Care Provider Failure and Support

Given the high level of care provider failure reported in the formal study, I asked two questions in the Changing Depression Survey regarding who respondents felt were most and least helpful in getting them help for PPD. The first question, Who was MOST responsible for your getting help for postpartum depression (PPD)?, yielded strong data regarding women's perception of self as an agent in accessing care for PPD. Given six options (see Figure 7), 65.4% (n = 318) selected "Self"; 23.0% (n = 112) selected "Partner"; 16.9% (n= 82) selected "Family Member"; 11.7% (n=57) selected "Medical Care Provider"; 8.8% (n= 55) selected "Other (Friend),"and only 6.6% (n=32) selected "Therapist." Figure 7 represents the findings.

When asked, Who was LEAST helpful in getting you help for postpartum depression (PPD)?, the majority of women (n=210; 43.2%) reported Medical Care Providers (OB/GYN, Midwife, General, or Family Physician) as least helpful; 21% (n=105) reported family members as least helpful; 20.6% (n=100) reported that their partner was least helpful; 19.3 % (n=93) reported Self as least helpful; and 6.8% (n=33) reported therapist as least helpful (see Figure 8).

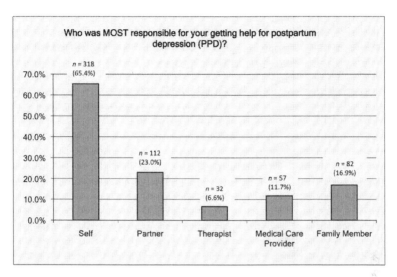

Figure 7. Changing Depression Survey: Who Was Most Helpful?

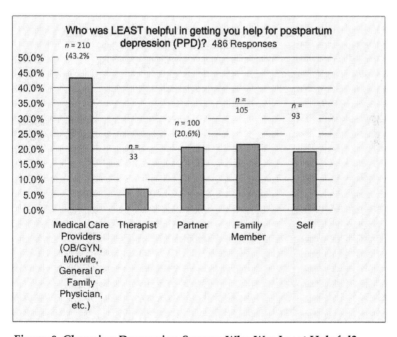

Figure 8. Changing Depression Survey: Who Was Least Helpful?

Clearly, the data in my formal study and the data gathered here strongly suggest a lack of provider support in helping women who suffer with PPD. Again, understanding this informal survey was just that—informal and a survey. Nonetheless, a large number of respondents gives strength to the suggestion that medical, obstetric, and mental health providers are more frequently not helpful than they are helpful. Moreover, in contrast to the reports of women experiencing deficiencies in help-seeking behaviors, this data strongly suggests the opposite. The majority of women (n = 318) reported that they were the most helpful in getting themselves help for PPD. Again, what are we missing? The gaps in direct service from provider to patient, and the lack of understanding as to the strength and resourcefulness of women present interesting opportunities to re-view standard practices of care, and re-search the inner potential of women who experience mood or anxiety disorders postpartum.

Additional Interview Notes

Throughout the writing of the book, I continued to gather data as grounded theory asserts. I recruited another sample of women who self-identified as having had PPD, and having changed as a result of it. The recruitment took place through the internet, via social media. Ten women agreed, and informed consent was obtained for all women with regards to using their stories in this book as part of my ongoing research. I asked women to answer three questions, selected for descriptive, explanatory, and exploratory inquiry (Marshall & Rossman, 2006).

1. *How would you describe your experience of postpartum depression (PPD)?*

2. *How did PPD change you?*

3. *How do you experience the transformation currently?*

I did not describe my research findings, nor did I define change or transformation. Eight of the 10 women described the experience of PPD and the process of transformation in the same ways observed in the formal study. Women described being unprepared for the onset of symptoms and experienced extreme distress about the symptoms. Women reported running the gauntlet of provider and system failures to get adequate treatment, and struggling to survive through severe symptoms of depression that included suicidal ideation and intrusive thoughts.

For two of the 10, Catherine and Leah, the change that occurred was not positive. Sharing their stories is a critical reminder that not every woman who develops PPD experiences positive growth.

Catherine's Story

How would you describe your experience of postpartum depression (PPD)?

I gave birth to my incredibly healthy son 1/3/2013. I am a first-time mom. My labour wasn't that bad, thanks to epidural, but my recovery was long and painful. I felt paralyzed in the beginning. For the first three weeks, my mother came and stayed to help out, and I barely wanted to spend time with my son. My husband and mother were doing most of the caregiving and I felt guilty about that. I struggled and hated breastfeeding, and by May, I gave up and started feeding my son formula and I hoped that being freed from breastfeeding would make me feel better, and that I would finally have the wherewithal to finally go out with my son and take him places. But since then, I have yet to take my son out of my house by myself. I never leave the house, and whenever I see my fellow mommy friends posting Facebook updates of themselves with their babies going out to cafes or having fun, I feel envious. I have a bad habit of comparing myself to others.

How did PPD change you?

I used to love animals. Cats especially. I used to love food, cooking, having fun in general. None of that exists anymore.

How do you experience the transformation currently?

I am taking Zoloft and I have a therapist who I am in contact with via email, so I am getting treatment. But I've only started treatment a month ago. I'm far from feeling normal, and I don't expect to feel better overnight. But I have been able to think more clearly, and I am slowly learning how to address my problems.

Leah's Story

How would you describe your experience of postpartum depression (PPD)?

Horrible, life changing, unexpected, miserable. I felt like I was in a black hole that I would never get out of. I felt like a terrible mother, wife, person. I felt crazy. I felt sad. I felt anxious. I felt hopeless. I thought it would never end.

How did PPD change you?

It changed my outlook on having other children. The thought of having to go through what I went through again with another pregnancy or child scared me. It freaked me out. Even though I knew better, I did not want our daughter to be an only child. So when our daughter was 3, I got pregnant again and I totally freaked out. So stressed and worried, and depressed, and anxious that I miscarried a week later. And I was SO relieved. A year later, I got the bright idea that I could handle it again, so my husband and I tried again. And I got pregnant right away. And once again I immediately freaked, panicked, and fell into a deep depression. So I did what I felt was right at the time (and I still do, but it makes me sad at times), and I had an abortion. Me, a married mom of one. With my husband supporting me all the way. So PPD changed my life for life. And my daughter is now 17, and still is an only child.

234

How do you experience this transformation currently?

PPD robbed me of having another child. And I am still on Zoloft 17 years later. I can remember the PPD like it was yesterday. I have a beautiful daughter, a wonderful husband, but the PPD took something away from me that I will never get back.

Caroline's Story

How would you describe your experience of PPD?

The hardest experience I didn't realize I was having. I had PPD following the birth of my second child, and much of my realizations came in hindsight. I knew, on some level, that I was struggling, as did many of my friends and husband, but I did a really good job of wearing the "I'm fine" mask. I am a therapist, and felt I had to tools to "heal myself" on some days, and completely denied how much of a problem I was having the other days. Later, I realized that my PPD began in the hospital, and gradually worsened over a period of several months.

I never reached out for help. In my work now, helping others who are struggling with PMADs, I think my experience helps me decrease the shame about the difficulty of asking for help. I can say, "I get it," but I can also say that there is no special award at the end of the journey for those who trudge through on their own.

How did PPD change you?

I learned that it is OK to be vulnerable and to ask for help. I learned that hiding it is really not protecting anyone. I also learned who my real friends (and family) are, as most people do when they are going through a crisis. My experience also forced me to delve into my own family history of mental illness, and some healing was found by recognizing that my own mom went through a PMAD, as did her own mother. It helped me understand a bit more about my reluctance to have a girl (one of the factors that I believe contributed to my PPD), and that I had the power to break the cycle.

How do you experience the transformation currently?

I have done a lot of work on myself in regards to relationships. I am on a quest (yes, that sounds very dramatic) to be real about my relationship with my daughter, who is now 8, and the difficulties that my experiences have brought to that. I want to educate her as she gets older about mental health, and to not be ashamed if she struggles someday if or when she has children. In my work, I have built a practice helping women and couples who are building their families and encounter difficulties. Helping them through their journeys is one of the most rewarding things I have ever done, and I am lucky to do it every day!

Mandy's Story

How would you describe your experience of postpartum depression (PPD)?

It was awful. Fortunately, it was short, but it was acute and severe. The sadness and excessive worry began on postpartum day 3. I had some insomnia, irritability and intrusive thoughts. I reached out to my midwife, my therapist, a few friends, and a few family members. I started Zoloft on postpartum day 4. Even though the medication hadn't started to set in, I began feeling slightly better for the next few days.

However, on postpartum day 9, I became overwhelmed because my mother (who had been at the house helping) was going home, and my husband was returning to work. The intrusive thoughts came back and were very startling. I had no idea why I was having them. I was convinced that I was losing my mind. I thought I would feel better if I could sleep. I went to the ER hoping they could help me sleep. I explained my intrusive thoughts and how I feared they meant I was going to hurt my son or myself. I was put in a barren room that was guarded by a police officer. No one tried to help me or talk to me. A crisis counselor spoke to me for about 15 minutes and asked some questions. They just took my temperature and blood pressure a lot. I didn't sleep much because the police officer at my door was talking to all night to nurses and other staff members. I asked to go home, but they told me

I was very ill and in need of inpatient treatment. I didn't think that sounded right, but I was so worried about myself and aware that I was not well so I agreed to go to a psychiatric institution.

The hours I spent at the psychiatric institution were the worst 24 hours of my life. There was little therapy offered. The other patients there were completely zoned out, yelling, or behaving as if they were young children. I felt very alone, scared, and misunderstood. Luckily, a psychiatrist met with me and felt that I should go home. I returned home and stayed on the Zoloft (even though the psychiatrist had told me to stop taking it if I wanted to breastfeed). I slept a lot and had family support for a few weeks. I began feeling better immediately. The anxiety was still there, but it significantly decreased. By the time my son was 1 month old, I felt like I had pulled myself out of the incredibly dark and confusing hole in which I had fallen.

How did PPD change you?

Before having PPD, I had what I considered mild experiences with depression and anxiety. (I also had had an eating disorder and I had always known the root of the ED was in anxiety and depression.) But my PPD experience made me realize how powerful anxiety and depression can be (on everything—your physical self, spiritual self, ability to fulfill day-to-day responsibilities, ability to work to your full potential). I looked back at my life and realized how I had always had anxious tendencies. Knowing how devastating the anxiety was during the postpartum period, I wanted recovery from the anxiety even more than I had before. I read about chemical pathways in our brains and realized I wanted to stop the anxious pathways in my brain. So, in a way, the PPD taught me to take better care of myself.

I've also realized that I am smarter than I give myself credit for, I understand myself better than anyone else, and in my gut, I know what is right and best for me. I truly believe I did everything in my power to get help for an illness that too many women are afraid to speak about. However, the system failed me. The misunderstanding of my illness (PPA, PPD, and PPOCD–not psychosis, suicidal or homicidal–which is what I think the ER staff thought I had) was inexcusable. I've always been an over-achiever and I hold myself to high standards. In many aspects of my life, I am respected for my hard work and abilities. Yet I still have so many insecurities. The PPD experience has made me realize that I want to work on those insecurities. I want to believe in myself and stop seeking the approval of others. Likewise, the experience reminded me to accept myself for who I am and learn to live with "good enough" because striving for excellence in everything is a sure way back to illness for me.

My postpartum experience was so compelling that I wrote a book about the situation. After writing the book, I began blogging to share my story and promote my book. I'm so proud of myself. After being a mom, this is the biggest accomplishment of my life. So the PPD/PPA/PPOCD experience changed me in that way too, I suppose.

I think I have more gratitude due to the experience as well. I am thankful for my family support, my friends, and the professionals that were able to help me. I see such kindness and bravery in the women who advocate about this topic and I am overwhelmed with hope, gratitude, and a feeling of purpose when I read about other "warrior" moms. Having been in a depressive state, I am so thankful to not be there, to be able to enjoy a brisk fall day, my son's engaging personality, my husband's quirks, etc. Finally, I am thankful for my strength and way of dealing with this whole ordeal. I am thankful that somehow, I had the tools to get through the whole mess.

How do you experience the transformation currently?

I certainly have more knowledge than I used to have— knowledge about myself, about PMADs and about others. I am more aware of my perfectionist tendencies, so I try not to overcommit myself. I have more confidence in myself. I feel stronger. I feel compelled to tell my story and improve the resources for women struggling with a PMAD. I have such a desire to raise awareness that I get annoyed at the fact that I can't make this my #1 mission in life. If I had all the money in the world, I would quit my job and devote myself 100% to this cause. But then I remember the statement above: I am more aware of my perfectionist tendencies so I try not to overcommit myself.

Victoria's Story

Victoria (pseudonym) shared

My baby boy was born April 7th, 2013. I was happy he was here, but bewildered, and not sure what to do, as he is my first. We struggled with breastfeeding from the start. Everyone assured me we would be fine. But we weren't. I felt immense pressure to breastfeed, but I hated it, and due to the amount my child was crying (since in the end he wasn't getting that much from me). I found myself angry at my child. This tiny human was on me all the time, demanding more, and it was never enough. I thought I was doing it right. I had read all the books and watched all the videos, but lo and behold, he would constantly cry, wake up, and I was exhausted. I would say this definitely became the catalyst for developing postpartum depression and anxiety. When I put him to the breast, because of his poor latch, it was so painful, I cried. We realized later that because I was expecting pain, and getting more and more anxious about feeding him. I just never let down properly and all he was getting was foremilk. He cried all the time because he was so hungry, but I didn't know that. I was a new mum who was still getting the hang of this whole motherhood thing.

After I was away from breastfeeding, I didn't want to go back to it, but the guilt crept back in every time, and I knew I would "have" to give it a try sooner or later. I thought if maybe I got some better help that I would enjoy it more if we would be able to iron out the problems we had.

So, I saw a lactation consultant who had excellent ratings from other new mums, but to me, she seemed neither empathetic nor supportive. My husband came with me the first visit, to help ease my growing anxiety. She had me take fenugreek and watch Dr. Jack Newman breastfeeding videos, read up on some studies on breastfeeding, and come back in a week. It was even worse the next visit. She critiqued my techniques, said my breast pump wasn't good enough and that it seemed like I "didn't even want to attempt to breastfeed," compounding the guilt and shame even more. After both visits, I sat in my car and cried my eyes out with my son sitting in the backseat. I felt so alone. No one I knew formula-fed, and I already felt so isolated.

In the end, I gave up on breastfeeding and switched to formula. Suddenly, I had a full, happy baby that starting growing like a weed. Problem solved, right? Wrong. My anxiety crept up more and more. I began to worry about what would happen if I took him out in public and he cried. I felt people were staring at me, thinking I was a terrible mother for not being able to soothe her child. When

I was having a "good" day, and took him out in public, and the crying (or even just simple fussing) happened, I would melt down in a full panic attack. I would suddenly be drenched in sweat from head to toe. I couldn't find the nearest exit to the street and fresh air. I felt dizzy and sick, short of breath, my heart beating a mile a minute. I would get to the car somehow, strap him in to his car seat, both of us in full meltdown mode. I would be driving fast to get home, tears streaming down my face, feeling so completely out of control, but needing to get home as soon as possible in order to feel "safe."

I avoided going out. I paced the floors of my house with my baby. I felt like I was an animal in a cage, but didn't want to get out. I was afraid. If I did go out with my son, it would be something safe, like going for a walk in the neighborhood with my husband. That was it. Again, on those "good" days, I would sometimes go on a walk with a friend, but if he fussed on the walk, I retreated as politely as possible, afraid that my friends would see this "other side" of me. I was embarrassed that I was acting so strangely.

I would have horrible thoughts pop into my head at random times. Thinking about how I could hang myself, and how I would do it near the end of the day so my son would not be left alone in his crib for too long before my husband arrived home. I dreamed of running away, dropping him off at my mother's house and driving until I couldn't drive anymore. I worried about everything to do with my baby. What if I was so tired, I tripped over the cat while I was holding him, and he would fly through the air and hit the wall, exploding his head? Carrying him down a flight of carpeted stairs and slipping, him falling out of my arms and breaking his neck? Thoughts like this popping into my head almost EVERY SINGLE DAY.

At 8 weeks, my son went for his first set of shots, and the public health nurse gave me the PPD screening question-naire, the Edinburgh test. My score was through the roof. So she sent a referral for me to see a counselor that is a specialist in PPD disorders. I waited one month to get in to see her. Within that first visit, she felt that my disorder was more chemically based, and would probably benefit from counselling and a visit with a psychiatrist. She was not able to refer me to the psychiatrist who specializes in this, only my family doctor (who was on long-term dis-ability, so I was suddenly doctorless) or my midwife.

I took up the subject with my midwife at our final visit, and she said that the referral would go in, and likely, a wait of 6 to 8 weeks to see the psychiatrist. I braced myself for almost two more months of "hanging on" with what felt like just the tips of my fingertips.

Three more weeks passed. I had heard nothing from the psychiatrist's office—surely they'd received my referral and would be calling me with my appointment by now?

I just wanted a date—mark my calendar with a big red "X"—something that I could count down towards. Just hang on a little longer.

I saw my counselor again and she thought something was strange about the referral not going through. She found the number for the office for me, and I called the next day. They had never heard of me, had not received my referral. Once again, I was at square one, and needed help. I called my midwife to ask if it had gone in, and she left me a message saying it had. Somewhere along the way, it had fallen through the cracks. Whether it was my midwife, who had forgotten, or a problem with technology receiving it on the other end. Who knows? But the point was, I had to wait almost EIGHT weeks at this point, due to summer holidays.

My baby was now over 4 months old. I had been suffering like this for over 4 months. One morning, I could not get my son back to sleep. It was 4:30 or 5 in the morning and I was so, so tired. I felt like I was drifting out to sea. Those fingertips that had been keeping me on the ledge were bloodied and worn away, and I could not hang on one second longer. I was weeping, sobbing uncontrollably, swept away in another panic attack. My husband woke up and overheard me on the baby monitor, took the baby, and put his arms around both of us. We would figure something out, he said.

When he had put our son back to sleep, he came to bed and we talked about our game plan. He said that he could not bear to see me living like this for another day (bless his heart), and we had to take matters into our own hands. So he took the day off work, drove me to the emergency room, and I had myself checked in to the psych ward for observation and help. It was one of the scariest days of my life, sitting next to people with cuts up their arms, people without shoes because they would try and strangle themselves or someone else, people staring at the floor sadly looking at nothing, people with armed guards watching over them. Was I one of those people?

It took almost a full day, pacing around a psych ward, to be seen by a nurse, a medical doctor, and finally, a psychiatrist—who, coincidentally, was the psychiatrist I would have been waiting for months to see. She looked into my face and told me that I would be okay, and I cried with my head in my hands. She prescribed me medication for anxiety and for depression. When I left that ward with the sun on my face and a prescription in my hands, I took a breath of fresh air, and I felt like a weight had been lifted off my shoulders. I felt like I had done something in my fight. I felt like a warrior.

I recently had a defining moment in motherhood. I was watching my son go to town in his Jolly Jumper, having the best time ever, that I cried. I couldn't stop the tears flowing because this was the FIRST time since he was born—including right after his birth—that I cried tears of pure JOY. I held my head up and let those delicious tears spill down my face and neck and soaked it in, crying and laughing at once. This moment here, is what it was supposed to be like to be a mother, I thought. I will remember that moment forever.

Everything that has happened to me throughout my journey has completely changed me and who I am. It's made me bolder, and more honest. It's made me realize how strong I really am, and how brave I am. I want to fight for better care for every single mum who is having a tough time. I want to do more. I want to share my story to let them know they are not alone, and it is nothing to be embarrassed about. Not only that, but sharing my story makes me feel like I'm more in control of this disorder that tries to set me back every single day. But every day, I rise with the sun, look at the most beautiful faces in the world—my son's and my husband's—and I smile. I smile with gratitude, with love, and with joy.

References

Abramowitz, J. S., Schwartz, S. A., Moore, K. M., & Luenzmann, K. R. (2002). Obsessive-compulsive symptoms in pregnancy and the puerperium: A review of the literature. *Anxiety Disorders, 426*, 1-18.

Allens, N. B., & Badcock, P. B. (2003). The social risk hypothesis of depressed mood: Evolutionary, psychosocial, and neurobiological perspectives. *Psychological Bulletin, 129*(6), 887-913.

Alloy, L. B., & Abramson, L. Y. (1979). Judgment of contingency in depressed and nondepressed students: Sadder but wiser? *Journal of Experimental Psychology: General, 108*, 441-485.

Almond, P. (2009). Postnatal depression: A global public health perspective. *Perspectives in Public Health, 129*(5), 221-227.

American Psychiatric Association (APA). (1994). *Diagnostic and statistical manual of mental disorders* (3rd Ed.). Washington, DC: Author.

American Psychiatric Association (APA). (2000). *Diagnostic and statistical manual of mental disorders* (4th Ed., Text rev.). Arlington, VA: Author.

American Psychiatric Association (APA). (2013). *Diagnostic and statistical manual of mental disorders* (5th Ed). Arlington, VA: Author.

Andrews, P. W., & Thompson, J. A., Jr. (2009). The bright side of being blue: Depression as an adaptation for analyzing complex problems. *Psychological Review, 116*(3), 620-623.

Baker-Ericzen, M. J., Mueggenborg, M. G., Hartingan, P., Howard, N., & Wilke, T. (2008). Partnership for women's health: A new-age collaborative program for addressing maternal depression in the postpartum period. *Families, Systems, & Health, 26*, 30-43.

Baker-Ericzén, M. J., Connelly, C. D., Hazen, A. L., Dueñas, C., Landsverk, J. A., & Horwitz, S. M. (2012). A collaborative care telemedicine intervention to overcome treatment barriers for Latina women with depression during the perinatal period. *Families, Systems, & Health, 30*(3), 224-240.

Banti, S., Mauri, M., Oppo, A., Borri, C., Rambelli, C., Ramacciotti, D., . . . Cossano, G. B. (2011). From the third month of pregnancy to 1 year postpartum. Prevalence, incidence, recurrence, and new onset of depression. Results from the perinatal depression-research and screening unit study. *Comprehensive Psychiatry, 52*, 343-351.

Barkin, J. L., & Wisner, K. L. (2013). The role of maternal self-care in new motherhood. *Midwifery, 29*(9), 1050-1055.

Beck, C. (2001). Predictors of postpartum depression: An update. *Nursing Research, 50,* 275-285.

Beck, C. (2006). Postpartum depression: It isn't just the blues. *American Journal of Nursing, 106*(5), 40-50.

Beck, C., & Driscoll, J. (2006). *Postpartum mood and anxiety disorders: A clinician's guide.* Sudbury, MA: Jones & Bartlett.

Beck, C., & Gable, R. K. (2000). Postpartum Depression Screening Scale: Development and psychometric testing. *Nursing Research, 49,* 272-282.

Bener, A., Gerber, L. M., & Sheikh, J. (2012). Prevalence of psychiatric disorders and associated risk factors in women during their postpartum period: A major public health problem and global comparison. *International Journal of Women's Health, 4,* 191-200.

Bennett, S., & Indman, P. (2011). *Beyond the blues: Understanding and treating prenatal and postpartum depression & anxiety* (4th Rev. Ed.). San Jose, CA: Moodswings Press.

Bernstein, I. H., Rush, A. J., Yonkers, K., Carmody, T. J., Woo, A., McConnell, K., & Trivedi, M. H. (2008). Symptom features of postpartum depression: Are they distinct? *Depression and Anxiety, 25,* 20-26.

Bilszta, J., Ericksen, J., Buist, A., & Milgrom, J. (2005). Women's experience of postnatal depression-beliefs and attitudes as barriers to care. *Australian Journal of Advanced Nursing, 27*(3), 44-54.

Blenning, C., & Paladine, H. (2005). An approach to the postpartum office visit. *American Family Physician, 72*, 2491-2496.

Borjesson, K., Ruppert, S., & Bagedahl-Strindlund, M. (2005). A longitudinal study of psychiatric symptoms in primiparous women: Relation to personality disorders and sociodemographic factors. *Archives of Women's Mental Health, 8*(4), 232-242.

Borowsky, S. J., Rubenstein, L., Meredith, L. S., Camp, P., Jackson-Triche, M., & Wells, K. B. (2000). Who is at risk of non-detection of mental-health problems in primary care? *Journal of General Internal Medicine, 15*(6), 381-388.

Bowen, A., Stewart, N., Baetz, M., & Muhajarine, N. (2009). Antenatal depression in socially high-risk women in Canada. *Journal of Epidemiology & Community Health, 63*, 414-416.

Bowlby, J. (1980). *Attachment and loss.* New York Basic Books.

Braud, W., & Anderson, R. (1998). *Transpersonal research methods for the social sciences: Honoring human experience.* Thousand Oaks, CA: Sage.

Brennan, P. A., Hammen, C., Andersen, M. J., Bor, W., Najman, J. M., & Williams, G. M. (2000). Chronicity, severity, and timing of maternal depressive symptoms: Relationships with child outcomes at age 5. *Developmental Psychology, 36*(6), 759-766.

Breslau, J., Kendler, K. S., Su, M., Gaxiola-Aguilar, S., & Kessler, R. C. (2005). Lifetime risk and persistence of psychiatric disorders across ethnic groups in the United States. *Psychological Medicine, 35*(3), 317-327.

Bruce, F., Berg, C., Hornbrook, M., Whitlock, E., Callaghan, M., Bachman, D., . . . Dietz, P. (2008). Maternal morbidity rates in a managed care population. *Journal of Obstetrics and Gynecology, 111*(5), 1089-1095.

Campbell, S. B., Matestic, P., von Stauffenberg, C., Mohan, R., & Kirchner, T. (2007). Trajectories of maternal depressive symptoms, maternal sensitivity, and children's functioning at school entry. *Developmental Psychology, 43*, 1202-1215.

Campbell, S. B., Morgan-Lopez, A. A., Cox, M. J., & McLoyd, V. C. (2009). A latent class analysis of maternal depressive symptoms over 12 years and offspring adjustment in adolescence. *Journal of Abnormal Psychology, 118*, 479-493.

Cerda, G. (2003, September). *A case for integrated mental health services for mother and child.* Paper presented at the National Center of Leadership in Academic Medicine, San Diego, CA.

Chang, J., Berg, C., Saltzman, L., & Herndon, J. (2005). Homicide: A leading cause of injury and deaths among pregnant and postpartum women in the United States, 1991-1999. *American Journal of Public Health, 95,* 471-477.

Chaudron, L. (2005). Self-recognition of and provider response to maternal depressive symptoms in low-income Hispanic women. *Journal of Women's Health, 14*(4), 331-338.

Chaudron, L., Kitzman, H. J., Peifer, K. L., Morrow, S., Perez, L. M., & Newman, M. C. (2005). Prevalence of maternal depressive symptoms in low-income Hispanic women. *Journal of Clinical Psychiatry, 66*(4), 418-423.

Chaudron, L., Klein, M., Remington, P., Palta, M., Allen, C., & Essex, M, (2001). Prodromes, predictors, and incidence of postpartum depression. *Psychosomatic Obstetrics & Gynecology, 22,* 103-112.

Cooper, L. A., Gonzales, J. J., Gallo, J. J., Rost, K. M., Meredith, L. S., Rubenstein, L. V., & Ford, D. E. (2003). The acceptability of treatment for depression among African-   American, Hispanic, and white primary care patients. *Medical Care, 41*(4), 479-489.

Copersino, M., Jones, H., Tuten, M., & Svikis, D. S. (2005). Suicidal ideation among drug-dependent treatment-seeking inner-city women. *Journal of Maintenance & Addiction, 3,* 53-64.

Cox, J. L., Holden, J. M., & Sagovsky, R. (1987). Detection of postnatal depression: Development of the 10-item Edinburgh Postnatal Depression Scale. *British Journal of Psychiatry, 150,* 782-786.

Creswell, J. W. (2009). *Research design: Qualitative, quantitative, and mixed methods approaches* (3rd Ed.). Thousand Oaks: Sage.

Darwin, C. (1872). *The expression of the emotions in man and animals.* London: John Murray.

Dennis, C-L., & Chung-Lee, L. (2006). Postpartum depression help-seeking barriers and maternal treatment preferences: A qualitative systematic review. *Birth, 33*(4), 323-331.

Diala, C. C., Muntaner, C., Walrath, C., Nickerson, K., LaVeist, T., & Leaf, P. (2001). Racial/ethnic differences in attitudes toward seeking professional mental health services. *American Journal of Public Health, 91*(5), 805-807.

Eberhard-Gran, M., Garthus-Nigel, S., Garthus-Nigel, K., & Eskild, A. (2010). Postnatal care: A cross-cultural and historical perspective. *Archives of Women's Mental Health, 6,* 459-466.

Figley, C. R. (1978). *Stress disorders among Vietnam veterans.* New York: Brunner/Mazel.

Fisher, J., Cabral de Mello, M., Patel, V., Rahman, A., Tran, T., Holton, S., & Homes, W. (2012). Prevalence and determinants of common perinatal mental disorders in women in low- and lower-middle-income countries: A systematic review. *Bulletin of World Health Organization, 90,* 139-149G.

Forman, D. N., Videbech, P., Hedegaard, M., Salvig, J. D., & Secher, N. J. (2000). Postpartum depression: Identification of women at risk. *British Journal of Obstetrics & Gynecology, 107,* 1210-1217.

Frankl, V. E. (1959). *Man's search for meaning.* New York: Pocket Books.

Franko, D. L., Blais, M. A., Becker, A. E., Delinsky, S. S., Greenwood, D. N., & Flores, A. T. (2001). Pregnancy complications and neonatal outcomes in women with eating disorders. *American Journal of Psychiatry, 158,* 1461-1466.

Gavin, N., Gaynes, B., Lohr, K., Meltzer-Brody, S., Garlehner, G., & Swinson, T. (2005). Perinatal depression: A systematic review of prevalence and incidence. *American Journal of Obstetrics and Gynecology, 106*(5, Pt. 1), 1071-1083.

Gaynes, B., Gavin, N., Meltzer-Brody, S., Lohr, K., Swinson, T., Gartlehner, G., & Miller, W. (2005). *Perinatal depression: Prevalence, screening accuracy, and screening outcomes: Summary, evidence report, and technology assessment* (No. 119). Rockville, MD: Agency for Healthcare Research & Quality.

Gold, K., & Marcus, S. (2008). Effect of maternal mental illness on pregnancy. *Expert Review of Obstetrics & Gynecology, 3*(3), 391-401.

Goodman, J. (2009). Women's attitudes, preferences, and perceived barriers to treatment for perinatal depression. *Birth, 36*(1), 60-69.

Goodman, S. H., & Dimidjian, S. (2012). The developmental psychopathology of perinatal depression: Implications for psychosocial treatment development and delivery in pregnancy. *Canadian Journal of Psychiatry, 57*(9), 530-536.

Goodman, S. H., & Tully, E. C. (2009). Recurrence of depression during pregnancy: Psychosocial and personal functioning correlates. *Depression and Anxiety, 26*(6), 557-567.

Hagen, E. H. (2011). Evolutionary theories of depression: A critical review. *Canadian Journal of Psychiatry/Revue Canadienne de Psychiatrie, 56*(12), 716-726.

Halligan, S. L., Murray, L., Martins, C., & Cooper, P. J. (2007). Maternal depression and psychiatric outcomes in adolescent offspring: A 13-year longitudinal study. *Journal of Affective Disorders, 97*(1), 145-154.

Hammen, C. (2005). Stress and depression. *Annual Review of Clinical Psychology, 1,* 293-319.

Hanley, J. (2009). *Perinatal mental health: A guide for health professionals and users.* West Sussex, England: John Wiley & Sons.

Harlow, B., Vitonis, A., Sparen, P., Cnattinguis, S., Joffe, H., & Hultman, C. (2007). Incidence of hospitalization for postpartum psychotic and bipolar episodes in women with and without prior pre-pregnancy or prenatal psychiatric hospitalizations. *Archives of General Psychiatry, 64*(1), 42-48.

Hay, D. F., Pawlby, S., Waters, C. S., & Sharp, D. (2008). Antepartum and postpartum exposure to maternal depression: Different effects on different adolescent outcomes. *Journal of Child Psychology and Psychiatry, 49*(10), 1079-1088.

Hayes-Bautista, D. E., Hsu, P., Perez, A., & Kahramanian, M. I. (2003). *The Latino majority has emerged: Latinos comprise more than 50 percent of all births in California.* Retrieved from http://cesla.med.ucla.edu/html/pdf/majority.pdf

Henry, A. L., Beach, A. J., Stowe, Z. N., & Newport, D. J. (2004). The fetus and maternal depression: Implications for antenatal treatment guidelines. *Clinical Obstetrics & Gynecology, 47*(3), 535-546.

Henshaw, C. (2007). Maternal suicide. In M. Pawson & J. Cockburn (Eds.), *Psychological challenges in obstetrics and gynecology: The clinical management* (pp. 157-164). London: Springer.

Heron, J., O'Connor, T. G., Evans, J., Golding, J., & Glover, V. (2004). The course of anxiety and depression through pregnancy and the postpartum in a community sample. *Journal of Affective Disorders, 80,* 65-73.

Holmes, T. H., & Rahe, R. H. (1967). The social readjustment rating scale. *Journal of Psychosomatic Research, 11*, 213-218.

Holzman, C., Eyster, J., Tiedje, L. B., Roman, L. A., Seagull, E., & Rahbar, M. H. (2006). A life course perspective on depressive symptoms in mid-pregnancy. *Journal of Maternal & Child Health, 10*(2), 127-138.

Horowitz, M. (1976). *Stress response syndromes*. New York, NY: Jason Aronson.

Howard, L. M., Flach, C., Mehay, A., Sharp, D., & Tylee, A. (2011). The prevalence of suicidal ideation identified by the Edinburgh Postnatal Depression Scale in postpartum women in primary care: Findings from the RESPOND trial. *BMC Pregnancy & Childbirth, 11*, 57.

Howell, E. A., Mora, P. A., Horowitz, C. R., & Leventhal, H. (2005). Racial and ethnic differences associated with early postpartum depressive symptoms. *Obstetrics and Gynecology, 105*, 1442-1450.

Institute of Medicine. (2011, March 15). *Leading health indicators for Healthy People 2020*: Retrieved from http://iom.edu/Reports/2011/Leading-Health-Indicators-for-Healthy-People-2020.aspx

Jackson, P. B., & Williams, D. R. (2006). Culture, race/ethnicity, and depression. In C. L. Keyes, & S. H. Goodman (Eds.), *Women and depression: A handbook for the social, behavioral, and biomedical sciences* (pp. 328-359). New York: Cambridge University Press.

Jesse, D. E., & Swanson, M. S. (2007). Risks and resources associated with antepartum risk for depression among rural southern women. *Nursing Research, 56*(6), 378-386.

Jesse, D. E., Walcott-McQuigg, J., Mariella, A., & Swanson, M. S. (2005). Risks and protective factors associated with symptoms of depression in low-income African American and Caucasian women during pregnancy. *Journal of Midwifery & Women's Health, 50*(5), 405-410.

Johnstone, S. J., Boyce, P. M., Hickey, A. R., Morris-Yatees, A. D., & Harris, M. G. (2001). Obstetric risk factors for postnatal depression in urban and rural community samples. *Australian and New Zealand Journal of Psychiatry, 35*, 69-74.

Josefsson, A., Angelsioo, L., Berg, G., Ekstrom, C. M., Gunnervik, C., & Nordin, C. (2002). Obstetric, somatic, and demographic risk factors for postpartum depressive symptoms. *Obstetrics and Gynecology, 99*, 223-228.

Joseph, G. (2009). New president to focus on postpartum depression. *ACOG Today, 53*(6), 1-3.

Katz, L. D. (2013). Pleasure. In N. Zalta (Ed.), *The stanford encyclopedia of philosophy* (para. 1). Retrieved from http://plato.stanford.edu/archives/spr2013/entries/pleasure

Kendall-Tackett, K. (2010). *Depression in new mothers: Causes, consequences, and treatment alternatives* (2nd Ed.). London: Routledge.

Kessler, R. (2003). Epidemiology of women and depression. *Journal of Affective Disorders, 74*(1), 5-13.

Keyes, C., & Goodman, S. (2006). *Women and depression: A handbook for the social, behavioral, and biomedical sciences.* New York: Cambridge University Press.

Kim-Cohen, J., Moffitt, T. E., Taylor, A., Pawlby, S. J., & Caspi, A. (2005). Maternal depression and children's antisocial behavior: Nature and nurture effects. *Archives of General Psychiatry, 62*(2), 173-181.

Knitzer, J., Theberge, S., & Johnson, K. (2008). *Reducing maternal depression and its impact on young children: Toward a responsive early childhood policy framework.* New York: National Center for Children in Poverty.

Kop, W. J., & Gottdiener, J. S. (2005). The role of immune system parameters in the relationship between depression and coronary artery disease. *Psychosomatic Medicine, 67*(Suppl. 1), S37-S41.

Kumar, R. (1994). Postnatal mental illness: A transcultural perspective. *Social Psychiatry and Psychiatric Epidemiology, 29,* 250-264.

Lancaster, C. A., Gold, K. J., Flynn, H. A., Yoo, H., Marcus, S. M., & Davis, M. M. (2010). Risk factors for depressive symptoms during pregnancy: A systematic review. *American Journal of Obstetrics & Gynecology, 202*(1), 5-14.

Lee, A. M., Lam, S. K., Mun Lau, S. M., Chong, C. S., Chui, H. W., & Fong, D. Y. (2007). Prevalence, course, and risk factors for antenatal anxiety and depression. *Obstetrics & Gynecology, 110*(5), 1102-1112.

Leigh, B., & Milgrom, J. (2008). Risk factors for antenatal depression, postnatal depression and parenting stress. *BMC Psychiatry, 8,* 11.

Lewis, A. J. (1934). Melancholia: A clinical survey of depressive states. *British Journal of Psychiatry, 80*(329), 277-378.

Lewis, G. (2007). The Confidential Enquiry into Maternal and Child Health (CEMACH). *Saving Mothers' Lives: Reviewing maternal deaths to make motherhood safer–2003–2005. The seventh report on confidential enquiries into maternal deaths in the United Kingdom.* London: CEMACH.

Lewis, G., & Drife, J. (2004). *Why mothers die: 2000-2002. The sixth report of confidential enquiries into maternal deaths in the United Kingdom.* London: CEMACH.

Lindahl, V., Pearson, J., & Colpe, L. (2005). Prevalence of suicidality during pregnancy and postpartum. *Archives of Women's Mental Health, 8*, 77-87.

Linley, P. A., & Joseph, S. (2004). Positive change processes following trauma and adversity. A review of the empirical literature. *Journal of Traumatic Stress, 17*, 11-12.

Maloney, J. (1952). Postpartum depression or third day depression following childbirth. *New Orleans Child Parent Digest, 6*, 20-32.

Marcus, S., Flynn, H., Blow, F., & Barry, K. (2003). Depressive symptoms among pregnant women screened in obstetrics settings. *Journal of Women's Mental Health (Larchmont), 14*(4), 373-380.

Marshall, C., & Rossman, G. B. (2011). *Designing qualitative research* (5th ed.). Thousand Oaks, CA: Sage.

Maslow, A. H. (1969). Toward a humanistic biology. *American Psychologist, 24*(8), 724-735.

Matthey, S. (2008). Using the Edinburgh Postnatal Depression Scale to screen for anxiety disorders. *Depression and Anxiety, 25*, 926-931.

McGuire, T. G., Alegria, M., Cook, B. L., Wells, K. B., & Zaslavsky, A. M. (2006). Implementing the Institute of Medicine definition of disparities: An application to mental health care. *Health Services Research, 41*(5), 1979-2005.

Mental Health America, Substance Abuse, and Mental Health Services Administration. (2009). *Maternal depression making a difference through community action: A planning guide.* Washington, DC: Government Printing Office.

Miranda, J., & Cooper, L. A. (2004). Disparities in care for depression among primary care patients. *Journal of General Internal Medicine, 19*(2), 120-126.

Moore, A. (2008). Hedonism. In N. Zalta (Ed.), *The Stanford encyclopedia of philosophy.* Retrieved from http://plato.stanford.edu/archives/spr2013/entries/hedonism

Moore, M. T., & Fresco, D. M. (2007). Depressive realism and attributional style: Implications for individuals at risk for depression. *Behavior Therapy, 38*, 144-154.

Mora, P. A., Bennett, I. M., Ito, I. T., Mathew, L., Coyne, J. C., & Culhane, J. F. (2009). Distinct trajectories of perinatal depressive symptomatology: Evidence from growth mixture modeling. *American Journal of Epidemiology, 169*(1), 24-32.

Moses-Kolko, E., & Roth, E. K. (2004). Antepartum and postpartum depression: Healthy mom, healthy baby. *Journal of the American Medical Women's Association, 59*, 181-191.

Murray, L., Arteche, A., Fearson, P., Halligan, S., Goodyer, I., & Cooper, P. (2011). Maternal postnatal depression and the development of depression in offspring up to 16 years of age. *Journal of the American Academy of Child & Adolescent Psychiatry, 50*(5), 460-470.

Murray, L., Cooper, P., Creswell, C., Schofield, E., & Sack, C. (2007). Social phobia on mother-infant interactions and infant social responsiveness. *Journal of Child Psychology and Psychiatry, 48*(1), 45-52.

Nadeem, E., Lange, J. M., Eddge, D., Fongwa, T., & Miranda, J. (2007). Does stigma keep poor, young, immigrant, and U.S.-born Black and Latina women from seeking mental health care? *Psychiatric Services, 58*, 1547-1554.

Nunes, M. A., Ferri, C. P., Manzolli, P., Soares, R. M., Drehmer, M., Buss, C., . . . Schmidt, M. (2010). Nutrition, mental health and violence: From pregnancy to postpartum cohort of women attending primary care units in Southern Brazil-ECCAGE study. *BMC Psychiatry, 10*, 66.

Oakley, A. (1993). *Essays on women, medicine and health.* Oxford, England: Edinburgh University Press.

Oates, M. (2003). Suicide: The leading cause of maternal death. *British Journal of Psychiatry, 183*, 279-281.

O'Hara, M. W. (2009). Postpartum depression: What we know. *Journal of Clinical Psychology, 65*(12), 1258-1269.

O'Hara, M. W., & Gorman, L. L. (2004). Can postpartum depression be predicted? *Primary Psychiatry, 11*(3), 42-47

O'Hara, M. W., & Segre, L. S. (2008). Psychological disorder of pregnancy and the postpartum. In R. S. Gibbs, B. Y. Karlan, A. F. Naey, & I. Nygaard (Eds.), *Danforth's obstetrics and gynecology* (10th ed.). Philadelphia, PA: Lippincott, Williams, & Wilkins.

O'Hara, M. W., & Swain, A. M. (1996). Rates and risk of postpartum depression: A meta-analysis. *International Review of Psychiatry, 8,* 37-54.

Orr, S. T. (2004). Social support and pregnancy outcome: A review of the literature. *Clinical Obstetrics & Gynecology, 47*(4), 842-855.

Palladino, C. L., Singh, V., Campbell, J., Flynn, H., & Gold, K. J. (2011). Homicide and suicide during the perinatal period: Findings from the National Violent Death Reporting System. *Obstetrics & Gynecology, 118*(5), 1056-1063.

Paris, R., Bolton, R., & Weinberg, M. (2009). Postpartum depression, suicidality, and mother-infant interactions. *Archives of Women's Mental Health, 12,* 309–321.

Pascoe, J. M., Stolfi, A., & Ormond, M. B. (2006). Correlates of mothers' persistent depressive symptoms: A national study. *Journal of Pediatric Health Care, 20,* 261-269.

Perez-Rodriguez, M., Baca-Garcia, E., Oquendo, M., & Carlos, B. (2008). Ethnic differences in suicidal ideation and attempts. *Primary Psychiatry, 15,* 44-58.

Postpartum Support International. (2012). *U.S. legislative action: 2012.* Retrieved June 3, 2013, from http://www.postpartum. net/News-and-Events/Legislation.aspx

Preston, J., & Johnson, J. (2009). *Clinical psychopharmacology made ridiculously simple* (6th Ed.). Miami, FL: MedMaster.

Price, J., Gardner, R., & Wilson, D. R. (2007). Territory, rank, and mental health: The history of an idea. *Evolutionary Psychology, 5*(3), 531-554.

Price, J., Sloman, L., & Gardner, R. (1994). The social competition hypothesis of depression. *British Journal of Psychiatry, 164*(3), 309-315.

Rahman, A., Iqbal, Z., & Harrington, R. (2003). Life events, social support, and depression in childbirth: Perspectives from a rural community in the developing world. *Psychological Medicine, 33*(7), 1161-1167.

Records, K., & Rice, M. (2007). Psychosocial correlates of depression symptoms during the third trimester of pregnancy. *Journal of Obstetric and Gynecological Nursing, 36*(3), 231-242.

Rich-Edwards, J. W., Kleinman, K., Abrams, A., Harlow, B. L., McLaughlin, T. J., Joffe, H., & Gillman, M. W. (2006). Sociodemographic predictors of antenatal and postpartum depressive symptoms among women in a medical group practice. *Journal of Epidemiology & Community Health, 60*(3), 221-227.

Rosenberg, P. B., Mielke, M. M., Xue, Q. L., & Carlson, M. C. (2010). Depressive symptoms predict incident cognitive impairment in cognitive healthy older women. *American Journal of Geriatric Psychiatry, 18,* 204-211.

Ross, L., & Dennis, C. (2009). The prevalence of postpartum depression among women with substance use, an abuse history, or chronic illness: A systematic review. *Journal of Women's Mental Health, 18*(4), 475-486.

Rubertsson, C., Waldenstrom, U., & Wickberg, B. (2003). Depressive mood in early pregnancy: Prevalence and women at risk in a national Swedish sample. *Journal of Reproductive and Infant Psychology, 21*(2), 113-123.

Rumi, J. (2004). *The essential Rumi: New expanded edition* (C. Barks, Trans.). New York: Harper One.

Rudnicki, S. R., Graham, J. L., Habboushe, D. F., & Ross, R. D. (2001). Social support and avoidant coping: Correlates of depressed mood during pregnancy in minority women. *Women & Health, 34*(3), 19-34.

Saczynski, J. S., Beiser, A., Seshardi, S., Auerbach, S., Wolf, P. A., & Au, R. (2010). Depressive symptoms and risk of dementia: The Framingham Heart Study. *Neurology, 75,* 35-41.

Segre, L. S., O'Hara, M. W., Arndt, S., & Stuart, S. (2007). The prevalence of postpartum depression: The relative significance of three social status indices. *Social Psychiatry & Psychiatric Epidemiology, 42,* 316-321.

Segre, L. S., O'Hara, M. W., & Losch, M. E. (2006). Race/ethnicity and perinatal depressed mood. *Journal of Reproductive & Infant Psychology, 24*(2), 99-106.

Seligman, M. (1975). *Helplessness: On depression, development, and death.* San Francisco: W. H. Freeman.

Seligman, M., & Csikszentmihalyi, M. (2000). Positive psychology: An introduction. *American Psychologist, 55*(1), 5-14.

Skouteris, H., Wertheim, E. H., Rallis, S., Milgrom, J., & Paxton, S. J. (2009). Depression and anxiety through pregnancy and the early postpartum: An examination of prospective relationships. *Journal of Affective Disorders, 113*, 303-308.

Snyder, C. R., & Lopez, S. J. (Eds.). (2002). *Handbook of positive psychology.* New York: Oxford University Press.

Somerset, W., Newport, J., Ragan, K., & Stowe, Z. (2006). Depressive disorders in women: From menarche to beyond menopause. In C. L. Keyes, & S. H. Goodman (Eds.), *Women and depression: A handbook for the social, behavioral, and biomedical sciences* (pp. 62-88). New York: Cambridge University Press.

Tedeschi, R. G., & Calhoun, L. G. (1996). The Posttraumatic Growth Inventory: Measuring the positive legacy of trauma. *Journal of Traumatic Stress, 9*, 455-471.

Tedeschi, R. G., & Calhoun, L. G. (2004). Posttraumatic growth: Conceptual foundations and empirical evidence. *Psychological Inquiry, 15*(1), 1-18.

Tennants, C. (2002). Life events, stress, and depression: A review of recent findings. *Australian and New Zealand Journal of Psychiatry, 36*(2), 173-182.

Trevathan, W. (2010). *Ancient bodies, modern lives: How evolution has shaped women's health.* New York: Oxford University Press.

Triplett, K. N., Tedeschi, R. G., Cann, A., Calhoun, L. G., & Reeve, C. L. (2012). Posttraumatic growth, meaning in life, and life satisfaction in response to trauma. *Psychological Trauma: Theory, Research, Practice, and Policy, 4*(4), 400-410.

U.S. Census Bureau. (2004). *Current populations survey, annual social and economic supplement: Ethnicity and ancestry statistics branch, population division.* Retrieved from http://www.census.gov.

U.S. Centers for Disease Control and Prevention. (2008). Prevalence of self-reported postpartum depressive symptoms in 17 states, 2004-2005. *MMWR Morbidity and Mortality Weekly Report, 57*(14), 361-366.

U.S. Centers for Disease Control. (2009). *HIV Surveillance Report, 21.* Retrieved from http://www.cdc.gov/hiv/topics/surveillance/resources/reports

U.S. Department of Health and Human Services. (n.d.). *Healthy people 2020: Determinants of health.* Retrieved from http://www.healthypeople.gov/2020/about/DOHabout.aspx

Vega, W. A., Kolody, B., & Aguilar-Gaxiola, S. (2001). Help seeking for mental health problems among Mexican Americans. *Journal of Immigrant Health, 3,* 133-140.

Vesga-Lopez, O., Blanco, C., Keyes, K., Olfson, M., Grant, B., & Hasin, D. (2008). Psychiatric disorders in pregnant and postpartum women in the United States. *Archives of General Psychiatry, 65,* 805-815.

Wan, E. Y., Moyer, C. A., Harlow, S. D., Fan, Z., Jie, Y., & Yang, H. (2009). Postpartum depression and traditional postpartum care in China: Role of *zuoyuezi*. *International Journal of Gynecology and Obstetrics, 104,* 209-213.

Wang, P. S., Berglund, P., Olfson, M., Pincus, H. A., Wells, K. B., & Kessler, R. C. (2005). Failure and delay in initial treatment contact after first onset of mental disorders in the National Comorbidity Survey Replication. *Archives of General Psychiatry, 62*(6), 603-613.

Westdahl, C., Milan, S., Magriples, U., Kershaw, T., Rising, S., & Ickovics, J. (2007). Social support and social conflict as predictors of prenatal depression. *Obstetrics and Gynecology, 110*(1), 134-140.

Wilson, R. S., Hoganson, G. M., Rajan, K. B., Barnes, L. L., Mendes de Leon, C. F., & Evans, D. A. (2010). Temporal course of depressive symptoms during the development of Alzheimer's disease. *Neurology, 75,* 21-26.

Wisner, K., Perel, J., Findling, R., & Hinnes, R. (2001). Prevention of recurrent postpartum depression: A randomized clinical trial. *Journal of Clinical Psychiatry, 62*(2), 82-86.

Wisner, K., Sit, D. Y., McShea, M. C., Rizzo, D. M., Zoretich, R. A., Hughes, C. L., . . . Hanusa, B.H. (2013). Onset timing, thoughts of self-harm, and diagnoses in postpartum women with screen-positive depression findings. *Journal of the American Medical Association/Psychiatry, 70*(5), 490-498.

Witt, W., DeLeire, T., Hagen, E., Wichmann, M., Wisk, L., Spear, H., . . . Hampton, J. (2010). The prevalence and determinants of antepartum mental health problems among women in the USA: A nationally representative population-based study. *Archives of Women's Mental Health, 13*, 425-437.

Wolf, A. W., De Andraca, I., & Lozoff, B. (2002). Maternal depression in three Latin American samples. *Social Psychiatry & Psychiatric Epidemiology, 37*, 169-176.

World Health Organization (WHO). (1992). *The ICD-10 Classification of Mental and Behavioural Disorders: Clinical descriptions and diagnostic guidelines*. Geneva: Author.

World Health Organization (WHO). (2001). *The world health report 2001, mental Health: New understanding. New hope*. Geneva: Author.

World Health Organization (WHO). (2003). *Managing complications in pregnancy and childbirth: A guide for midwives and doctors*. Retrieved from http://www.who.int/maternal_child_adolescent/documents/9241545879/en/

Index

D

E

L

M

N

O

Made in the USA
San Bernardino, CA
27 February 2017